AN UPDATE OF DENTAL IMPLANTOLOGY AND BIOMATERIAL

Edited by **Mazen Ahmad Almasri**

An Update of Dental Implantology and Biomaterial
http://dx.doi.org/10.5772/intechopen.73818
Edited by Mazen Ahmad Almasri

Contributors

Dalia Khalil, Margareta Hultin, Belir Atalay, W. Keung Leung, Wai Kan Andy Yeung, In Woong Um, Young-Kyun Kim, Pil-Young Yun, Zi-Yu Yan, Yu-Mi Kim, Pınar Gültekin, Adnan Kose, Deniz Sen

First published in London, United Kingdom, 2019 by IntechOpen
IntechOpen is the global imprint of INTECHOPEN LIMITED, registered in England and Wales, registration number: 11086078, The Shard, 25th floor, 32 London Bridge Street
London, SE19SG – United Kingdom
Printed in Croatia

British Library Cataloguing-in-Publication Data
A catalogue record for this book is available from the British Library

Additional hard copies can be obtained from orders@intechopen.com

An Update of Dental Implantology and Biomaterial, Edited by Mazen Ahmad Almasri
p. cm.
Print ISBN 978-1-78984-992-9
Online ISBN 978-1-78984-993-6

For EU product safety concerns:
IN TECH d.o.o., Prolaz Marije Krucifikse Kozulić 3, 51000 Rijeka, Croatia,
info@intechopen.com or visit our website at intechopen.com.

Meet the editor

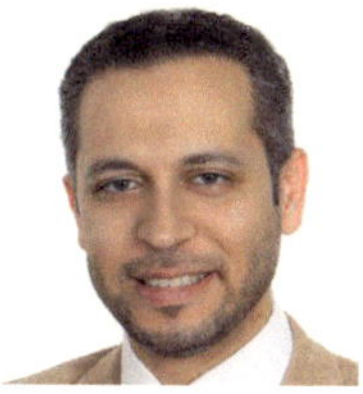

Dr. Mazen Ahmad Almasri is an associate professor and consultant of oral maxillofacial surgery (OMFS) at the Faculty of Dentistry in King Abdulaziz University (KAU), Jeddah City, Saudi Arabia. He graduated from KAU back in 2002 and went to McGill University (Montreal, Quebec, Canada) in 2005 for training and specialization in the field of OMFS, reconstruction, and dental implantology. Dr. Almasri succeeded in the residency training program, the fellowship of reconstruction and implantology, and the Masters of Dental Science degree. Thereafter, he became an active Fellow of the Royal College of Dentists of Canada (2009) and an active diplomat of the American Board of Oral Maxillofacial Surgery (2011). His passion for advancing clinical care and education has continued as a surgeon at KAU health center, an office clinical practitioner, a researcher, and an educator who believes in advancing the OMFS undergraduate and postgraduate programs.

Contents

Preface

Since the beginning of dental implant placement and the publication of the literature a dramatic advancement has taken place. In 2016 I had the honor to be part of the amazing team that participated in creating the textbook *Dental Implantology and Biomaterial*. More than 15 authors from more than seven countries from all over the globe participated in advancing the practice of implantology and research.

Today I am fortunate to be able to update the former textbook by discussing the challenges that implantologists face in a really busy practice.

As a surgeon who is usually asked to accomplish the reconstructive skeleton of the rehabilitation plan, questions like "Doc, I am in a hurry, how fast can you finish the treatment?" are becoming very common in practice these days This phenomenon goes hand in hand with people's current lifestyles. Although the advancement in reconstruction is appreciated, apparently it has not reached the limit of placing the factors of cost, time, and invasiveness into one location. I believe that cases should be treated and rehabilitated as soon as possible, with reasonable cost and feasible technicality so that clients can focus on their daily lives.

The solution to reconstruction is available but not always satisfactory. Free vascular flaps, bone morphogenic proteins, and stem cell treatment are hot topics of work and research; however, there are many drawbacks, starting with very high cost. Now, imagine if the procedure were to be repeated twice for the same patient.

One of the major areas that needs significant attention is the prognostication of factors relevant to dental care. Although it is clearly written in the literature, the importance of long-term success, up to 15 years post dental care, is clearly being omitted. I believe that if this would have been reported a lot of dental treatment plans would have been managed differently.

The same applies to the importance of not omitting regular checkups and taking panoramic dental radiographs, which could prevent the patient from developing major cysts or tumors. All this is the result of delaying dental treatment, which magnifies the number of defects, the type and volume of reconstruction work, and hence the cost.

With the incorporation of substantial subject matter, literature reviews, article analysis, up-to-date grafting carriers, immediate implantation tips, anterior implant cosmesis, and antibiotics for microbiota management, *An Update in Dental Implantology and Biomaterial* is the text that implantology specialists and trainees need to review. The three sections in the book start with a unique analysis of implantology literature, followed by a clinical procedures update, and finally restorations and the avoidance of peri-implantitis, the nightmare of any practitioner regardless of the specialty.

In King Abdulaziz University, multiple implant systems are being introduced for training and treatment. The staff have the luxury of comparing one system over the others. However, variable factors still need a lot of investigation, such as the technicality and grafting techniques. Such is the future of research in both Master's and PhD programs.

This book is aimed at students, residents, practitioners, and researchers in the field of implantology. It is expected to give them inspiration to understand how implantology is dynamically moving with novel ideas that are managing patients all over the world. And as the editor of the book, I thank all the contributors for their valuable work, effort, and patience. It has been a journey with many bumps and bruises, but finally it has come to fruition.

Acknowledgments

It is not uncommon that with every educational product, acknowledgments have their part in crediting the magnificent people whom I believe represent the backbone of dental education.

Therefore special gratitude goes to Professor Abdulrahman Bin Obaid Alyoubi, the respectful president of King Abdulaziz University, Jeddah, Saudi Arabia. Your extraordinary support for the medical institutes, the college, the community, and myself is highly appreciated. I have no better way to say thank you than with this book.

Also, special thanks go to the Dean of the Faculty of Dentistry, Professor Abdul Ghani Mira, and the vice deans, Rayyan Kayal, Ayman Aldharrab, Abdulelah Binmahfouz, and Sahar Bukhari. Warm appreciation goes to my colleagues and friends with whom I have been working closely to improve dental education: Dr. Ahmad Jan (former head of the OMFS Department), Dr. Maisa Alsebaie (head of the OMFS Department), and Dr. Abeer Alnuwaiser (chair of the internship training program).

During the time that I spent reviewing the details of this book, and assuring the addition of the new material, I would like to thank my family. Without their understanding and support, this would never have seen the light of day. Thank you, family and real friends, you have been always the power of prosperity.

Mazen A. J. Almasri, BDS, MSC, FRCD(c), Dipl ABOMS
Associate Professor/Consultant of Oral Maxillofacial Surgery
Department of OMFS, Faculty of Dentistry
King Abdulaziz University
Jeddah, Saudi Arabia

Section 1

Principles Before Dental Implant Placement

Chapter 1

The Growth of Dental Implant Literature from 1966 to 2016: A Bibliometric Analysis

Andy Wai Kan Yeung and Wai Keung Leung

Additional information is available at the end of the chapter

http://dx.doi.org/10.5772/intechopen.77223

Abstract

This bibliometric book chapter overviewed the dental implant literature from 1966 to 2016 via the Web of Science database. Articles and reviews published by 2016 on the topic of dental implants were identified and analyzed in terms of their authors, affiliations, countries/territories of the affiliations, journal title and journal category. The performance indices of the 10 journals with the highest numbers of dental implant publications were extracted from Journal Citation Reports. A total of 14,335 articles or reviews were published in 1081 academic journals, with majority (10,487; 73.2%) in dental journals. With 317,263 total citations, each publication was cited 22.1 times on average. About 10 journals accounted for 47.0% of total publications, five dedicated to dental implants. Performance indices of journals publishing dental implant manuscripts have been stable over the last decade. *Clinical Oral Implants Research* was the best performing journal among them in 2016.

Keywords: dental implants, bibliometric, impact factor, literature, publication

1. Introduction

Dental implantation is a treatment option for replacement of teeth missing due to disease or trauma. It has gained substantial support from oral healthcare providers and patients over the last two to three decades [1–3]. The popularity of this treatment modality has sparked numerous related research activities. Dental implant researches have assisted the evidence-based clinical practice of implant dentistry to a great extent. Multiple papers have critically and systematically reviewed the importance and relevancy of how such research results inform clinical practice [4–7]. These publications assessed the outcomes of researches that aimed at answering specific, important questions regarding dental implants and thus were expected to be read by a large audience. On the other hand, related bibliometrics could also be important to educators, researchers and healthcare workers in the dental field via analyzing the statistics of academic literature related to dental implantology. Such analyses have identified the most cited implant articles [8–10], popular implant research topics [11–13], highly cited topics [14], publication bias of implant journals [15, 16], and the distribution of evidence, which informs disease etiology, diagnosis, therapy and prognostic aspects relevant to dental implants [17]. They also can reveal the sources of past and recent research funding supporting the corresponding intellectual development [18, 19] and the quality assessment of implant case series [20] and systematic reviews/meta-analyses [21].

As more patients have become aware of dental implants as an option to replace missing teeth, the research fields of dental implantology have diversified and are receiving more attention. Usually the latest advancements in technology or treatment guidelines are published and distributed by academic journals. Since 94% of dental practitioners would place implants or refer patients with such treatment need to a colleague for the procedure, they benefit from keeping up to date on information on various aspects of dental implantation [3]. With the expansion of dental implant literature, it is crucial for practitioners and educators to quickly identify the leading literature from dental implant journals or other resources which would best potentially inform their practice and fulfill their continuous education needs. Past studies have tracked the time trends in journal performance indices, such as the Impact Factor, for selected journals in dentistry [22], public health [23], radiology [24] and medicine [25]. However, to the best knowledge of the authors, no published studies have investigated specifically the academic performance of journals dedicated to dental implants or which include many dental implant publications which inform the academic development concerning the field of implant dentistry.

Hence, this chapter aimed to track the dental implant publication counts over the last 50 years with considerations of annual trend and background publishing information, and then to identify the most productive journals and analyze their performance over the last decade. The implications of the findings were also discussed.

2. Study on dental implant literature

2.1. Literature search

The Thomson Reuters Web of Science database indexes academic publications and was the source of data for the study. The Web of Science database has been considered the golden standard to be used to extract and analyze bibliometric data of the existing scientific literature [26–30]. To identify appropriate keywords to perform a literature search, we searched the Medical Subject Headings (MeSH) library developed by the United States National Library of Medicine (NLM). The term "dental implantation" was used from 1966 to 1989 and was replaced by "dental implants" in 1990. In the Web of Science Core Collection database, we employed the term "dent* implant*" to search the "topic" of each record in the database. This would search for "dental implant" and its variants such as "dental implants" and "dental implantation" within the title, abstract and keywords of each indexed publication.

Publications from 2018 were excluded since the annual record was incomplete at the time of this study. Only articles and reviews were included.

The remaining records were described in terms of their annual trend of publications and citations. The publications were sorted by journal categories, journal titles, languages, countries/territories, organizations and authors. We analyzed the top 10 journals with the highest numbers of dental implant publications by examining their shares of the total publication counts. Further, we accessed the online version of Thomson Reuters Journal Citation Reports (JCR) to extract data of their bibliometric metrics, namely Impact Factor, Immediacy Index and Eigenfactor Score over the last decade from 2007 to 2016. The Impact Factor is a renowned metric, whereas the Immediacy Index indicates how fast articles in that journal are cited, and Eigenfactor Score is similar to Impact Factor but gives weighting to the citing journals and excludes the influence of self-citations. The bibliometric metrics of the top 10 dental journals with highest numbers of dental implant publications were tracked and examined.

The distributions of these dental implant publications among authors and journals were evaluated regarding whether they followed Price's law or Bradford's law, respectively. Price's law [31] states that half of the publications are written by a number of authors that equals to the square root of all authors. Meanwhile, Bradford's law [32] states that if journals are ranked according to their publication count and divided into three groups, with each group publishing one third of all papers, then the number of journals in each group should be in the ratio of $1/n/n^2$. In brief, a few core journals accounted for one third of all dental implant papers published, whereas many other journals each published a few only.

2.2. Survey outcome

The Web of Science Core Collection database was accessed on 6 March 2018. A search for the topic of "dent* implant*" in all years returned 17,954 records. After excluding records from 2017 and 2018, 16,002 records remained. Year 2017 was excluded because Impact Factor data was not yet available. After selecting only articles and reviews, 14,809 records remained. Publications within this pool were double-checked by the "Analyze Results" function to examine their document types, and subsequently 469 proceedings papers, 4 book chapters and one retracted publication were excluded. Finally, the search returned 14,335 documents, of which 13,283 were articles and 1052 were reviews.

2.2.1. Overview of the dental implant literature from 1966 to 2016

The first dental implant publication indexed in the Web of Science Core Collection was published in 1966. For the following two decades, the annual publication count was consistently below 15. The annual count reached 30 in 1990, and the dental implant literature has been steadily growing ever since, exceeding 100 publications in 1996 and 1000 in 2012. During the study period of 1966–2016, there were totally 14,335 dental implant publications that received 317,263 citations. On average, each publication was cited 22.1 times.

From 1966 to 2016, the 14,335 dental implant publications were recorded in 1081 academic journals distributed in 143 journal categories. There were 10,487 (73.2%) publications in

"Dentistry, Oral Surgery & Medicine" journals, 2765 (19.3%) in "Engineering, Biomedical", 1056 (7.4%) in "Materials Science, Biomaterials" and 901 (6.3%) in "Surgery". Note that these categories were not mutually exclusive since a journal could be assigned to multiple categories. For example, *Clinical Oral Implants Research* was indexed in the "Dentistry, Oral Surgery & Medicine" and "Engineering, Biomedical" categories and accounted for 57.3% (1584/2765) records of the latter category.

The 10 journals with the highest numbers of dental implant publications accounted for 47.0% of total publication count. Five of them were dedicated to dental implants, namely *International Journal of Oral & Maxillofacial Implants* (1621 publications; 11.3%), *Clinical Oral Implants Research* (1584; 11.1%), *Clinical Implant Dentistry and Related Research* (574; 4.0%) and *Implant Dentistry* (528; 3.7%) and *Journal of Oral Implantology* (418; 2.9%). The other five journals were not dedicated to dental implants but also belonged to the "Dentistry, Oral Surgery & Medicine" category (**Figure 1**). They were *Journal of Periodontology* (712; 5.0%), *Journal of Prosthetic Dentistry* (392; 2.7%), *Journal of Oral and Maxillofacial Surgery* (378; 2.6%) and *International Journal of Periodontics and Restorative Dentistry* (285; 2.0%) and *International Journal of Oral and Maxillofacial Surgery* (242; 1.7%). Three of these 10 journals each had 10% share of the total citation count (**Figure 1**). The first, second and last one-third of the articles and reviews were published by five, 32 and 1044 journals respectively (**Table 1**). If n = 32, the predicted distribution would be 1:32:1024. The actual distribution had more journals publishing the first one-third of all papers than predicted.

It is worth mentioning that some journals from the "Materials Science, Biomaterials" category represented a considerable share of the dental implant literature. *Biomaterials* had 148 (1.0%) publications. *Journal of Biomedical Materials Research* (published until 2002) had 95 (0.7%) publications, *Journal of Biomedical Materials Research Part A* (published since 2003) had 118 (0.8%) publications, and *Journal of Biomedical Materials Research Part B Applied Biomaterials* (published since 2003) had 103 (0.7%) publications, so in total 316 articles were published in the *Journal of Biomedical Materials* series. However, none of the biomaterials journals, when considered individually, had a larger total publication count than the tenth most prolific journal mentioned above (*International Journal of Oral and Maxillofacial Surgery*).

Most of the publications were in English (13,903; 97.0%), followed by German (166; 1.2%), French (58; 0.4%), Korean (57; 0.4%) and Spanish (37; 0.3%). All other languages had less than 30 indexed publications. Among the 109 countries/territories that the authors represented, the 10 countries with which the most institutions affiliated were the United States (3266; 22.8%), Italy (1633; 11.4%), Germany (1444; 10.1%), Brazil (1330; 9.3%), Sweden (876; 6.1%), Japan (817; 5.7%), Switzerland (813; 5.7%), South Korea (811; 5.7%), China (792; 5.5%), and Spain (775; 5.4%).

More than 5600 organizations have published on dental implants. The 10 most productive organizations were University of Gothenburg (510; 3.5%), University of Bern (357; 2.5%), São Paulo State University (356; 2.5%), University of Chieti-Pescara (351; 2.4%), University of São Paulo (343; 2.4%), University of Texas (280, 2.0%), University of Milan (262; 1.8%), New York University (261; 1.8%), University of Michigan (260; 1.8%), and Harvard University (228; 1.6%).

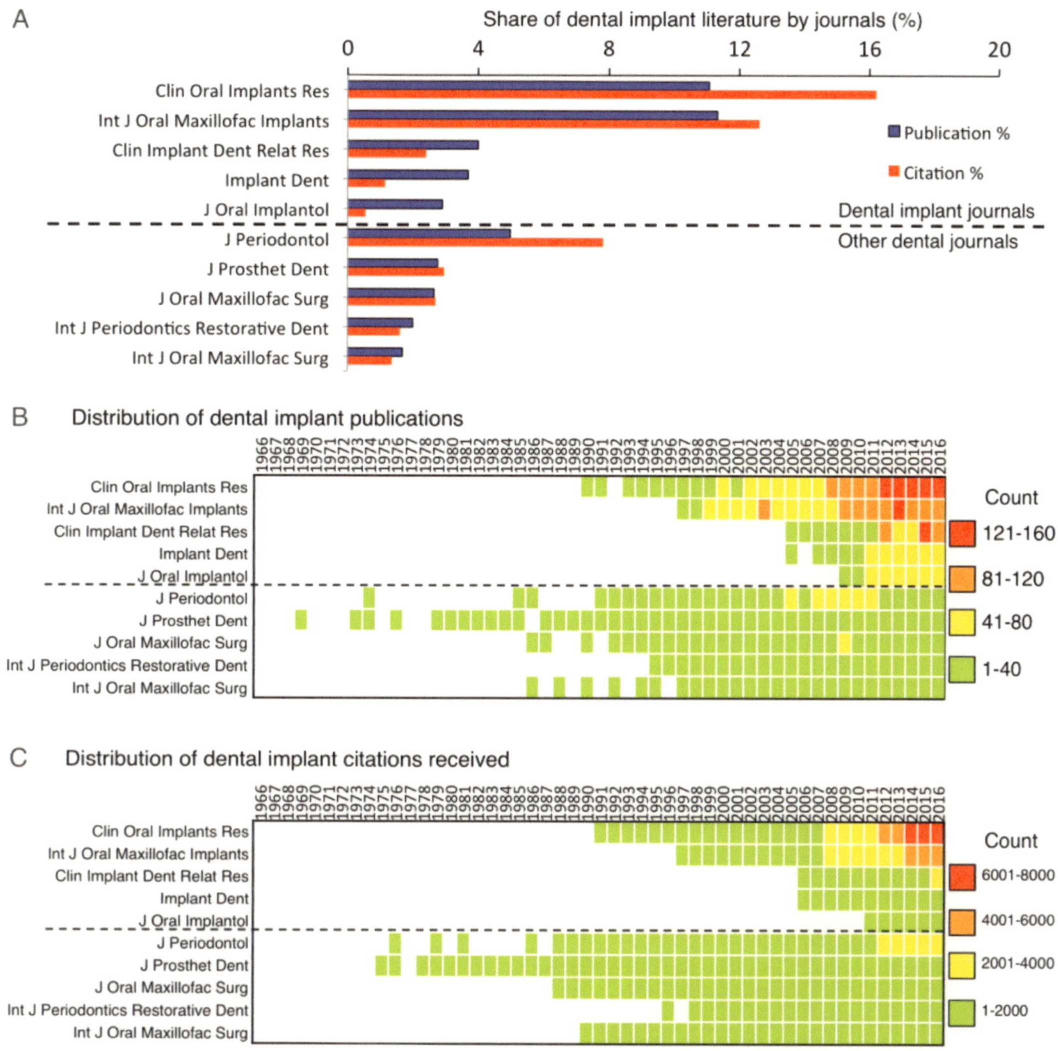

Figure 1. Time trend of annual publication counts for dental implant articles and reviews from 1966 to 2016 by the 10 most prolific journals which publish dental implant articles. (A) Publication and citation share of dental implant literature by journals; (B) distribution of dental implant publications over the survey period; (C) distribution of dental implant citation received over the survey period.

Over 28,800 authors have published on dental implants. Each author has published an averaged number of 2.3 papers (SD, 4.7). Over 80% of authors published either 1 (18,806; 65.2%) or 2 (4519; 15.7%) papers. The most prolific 164 authors have written 7641 articles or reviews, which roughly followed Price's law (170 authors should have written 7168 papers). The 10 most productive authors were Adriano Piattelli (251; 1.8%), Hom-Lay Wang (167; 1.2%), Marco Esposito (137; 1.0%), Niklaus P. Lang (121; 0.8%), Gerry M. Raghoebar (116; 0.8%), Paulo G. Coelho (104; 0.7%), Giovanna Iezzi (103; 0.7%), Daniel Buser (100; 0.7%), Antonio Scarano (96; 0.7%) and Henry J.A. Meijer (95; 0.6%).

	Journal	Pub count
Zone 1	International Journal of Oral Maxillofacial Implants	1621
	Clinical Oral Implants Research	1584
	Journal of Periodontology	712
	Clinical Implant Dentistry and Related Research	574
	Implant Dentistry	528
Zone 2	Journal of Oral Implantology	418
	Journal of Prosthetic Dentistry	392
	Journal of Oral and Maxillofacial Surgery	378
	International Journal of Periodontics Restorative Dentistry	285
	International Journal of Oral and Maxillofacial Surgery	242
	Journal of Clinical Periodontology	225
	Journal of Craniofacial Surgery	184
	European Journal of Oral Implantology	170
	International Journal of Prosthodontics	159
	Biomaterials	148
	Journal of Oral Rehabilitation	136
	Journal of Dental Research	129
	Journal of Prosthodontics Implant Esthetic and Reconstructive Dentistry	124
	Implantologie	122
	Journal of Biomedical Materials Research Part A	118
	Quintessence International	112
	Journal of Cranio Maxillofacial Surgery	110
	Medicina Oral Patologia Oral Y Cirugia Bucal	110
	Journal of Biomedical Materials Research Part B Applied Biomaterials	103
	Clinical Oral Investigations	98
	Journal of Materials Science Materials in Medicine	97
	Oral Surgery Oral Medicine Oral Pathology Oral Radiology and Endodontology	97
	Journal of Biomedical Materials Research	95
	Dental Materials	87
	Journal of The American Dental Association	86
	Dentomaxillofacial Radiology	85
	British Journal of Oral Maxillofacial Surgery	83
	Materials Science Engineering C Materials for Biological Applications	82
	Journal of Periodontal and Implant Science	80

Journal	Pub count
Clinical Advances in Periodontics	79
Journal of the Korean Association of Oral and Maxillofacial Surgeons	75
Journal of Advanced Prosthodontics	67

They are listed in descending order of implant original articles or reviews published from 1996 to 2016.

Table 1. Journals that published the first (zone 1, also known as core journals, as defined by Bradford's law) and second (zone 2) one-thirds of the publications.

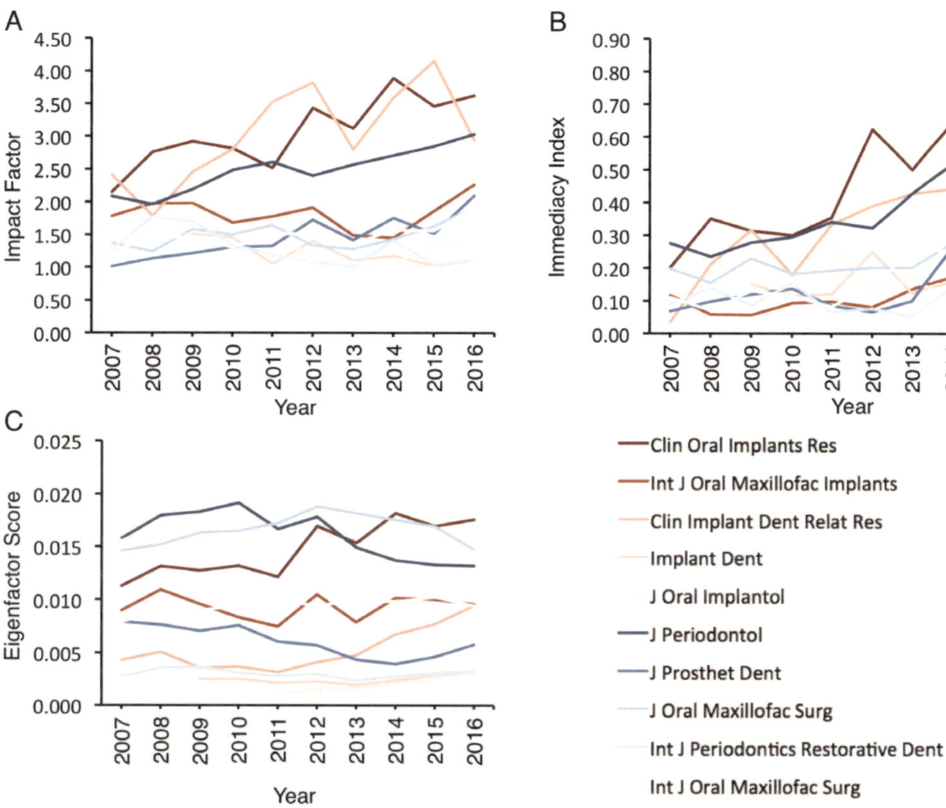

Figure 2. Performances of the 10 most prolific journals which published dental implant articles over the last decade (2007–2016) in terms of (A) impact factor, (B) immediacy index and (C) Eigenfactor score. The data lines for dental implant journals are in red, while those for other dental journals are in blue.

2.2.2. Performances of 10 selected journals in the last decade of 2007–2016

The top 10 journals with the highest numbers of dental implant publications were compared. The latest data published by JCR (bibliometric metrics in the year 2016) showed that *Clinical Oral Implants Research* had the highest Impact Factor (3.624; **Figure 2**), highest Immediacy Index (0.769; **Figure 2**) and highest Eigenfactor Score (0.0176; **Figure 2**) among the 10 journals with the highest numbers of dental implant publications. Over the entire period of 2007–2016, the Impact Factor of the journals stayed approximately within the range of 1–4. For an exploratory analysis, linear regressions have shown a significant linear increasing trend of the Impact Factor for most of these journals (except *International Journal of Oral and Maxillofacial Implants*, *Journal of Oral Implantology* and *International Journal of Periodontics Restorative Dentistry*) over the survey period. Similarly, most of these journals had a significant linear increasing trend of the Immediacy Index (except Implant Dentistry, *Journal of Oral Implantology* and *International Journal of Periodontics Restorative Dentistry*).

3. Discussion

Reported here is the first account that reviewed trends in the dental implant literature all the way from the 1960s to the present while simultaneously examining the bibliometric metrics of representative journals over the last decade. Since the early studies of dental implants were published half a century ago, nearly three quarters of the successive publications have been within dental journals. It has been suggested that the increase in dental implant publications in recent years can be attributed to the increased collaboration between authors, institutions and countries [12]. Given the substantial increase observed in the annual publication count of dental implant articles and reviews, it was demonstrated that dental implantology has emerged as an important research field in dentistry. The distribution of publications followed Price's law, implying that there are dominant authors who have strong contributions to the field. However, the distribution of publications showed more journals publishing the first one-third of all papers than predicted by Bradford's law, implying that readers should look for multiple journals instead of a single journal when they want to search for implant publications. Another implication is that no single journal is dominating the publishing market of dental implant papers as predicted by Bradford's law.

European scientists and clinicians were key players in dental implant research who were responsible for three fifths of the total publications from 1966 to 2016, and 5 of the 10 most productive organizations were in Europe. North America came in second, as it was responsible for one quarter of the publications and had three organizations in the top 10. Asia and South America were responsible for one fifth and one tenth of the publications respectively. Unlike Barão et al.'s [19] work, which classified the geographic origin of articles by the location of corresponding authors, the counts of geographic origin in this study were not mutually exclusive, and thus we could not directly compare the figures reported in the two studies. However, Barão et al. [19] reported that Europe accounted for nearly half of the articles published in five selected implant-related journals from 2005 to 2009, while North America and Asia accounted for one fifth each. These findings implied that the bulk of the dental implant researches were based in Europe, and they were consistent with the fact that major implant brands were based in Europe, such as Nobel Biocare (Zurich, Switzerland) and Straumann (Basel, Switzerland).

Russo et al. [17] reported that *Clinical Oral Implants Research*, *International Journal of Oral & Maxillofacial Implants*, *Journal of Prosthetic Dentistry* and *Journal of Oral & Maxillofacial Surgery* were the four most productive journals, accounting for nearly 50% of the dental implant papers published from 1994 to 1999. Our results confirmed that they were among the top 10 journals with the highest numbers of dental implant publications over the last 50 years. However, these four journals only accounted for 28% of the all-time implant publications included in our study. This difference may be considered in several aspects. First, there was a difference in search criteria. While Russo et al. [17] searched for English articles on human dental implants on MEDLINE database, we searched for all dental implant articles and reviews on the Web of Science database. Another important consideration was that recently introduced implant-specific journals might have taken a share, such as *Clinical Implant Dentistry and Related Research*, which started in 1999, and *European Journal of Oral Implantology*, which started in 2008. Meanwhile, Tarazona et al. [13] has evaluated implant literature contributed by Spanish researchers and concluded that the *Clinical Oral Implants Research* and *Medicina Oral Patologia Oral y Cirugia Bucal* were the most prolific journals. This has implied that certain journals may have a regional preference. In fact, the research topics or types of studies are also geographic dependent. A previous survey [19] has reported that clinical studies were mostly conducted by North American and European research teams supported by industrial funding, whereas the Asian and South American research teams were more focused on *in vitro* or animal studies supported by governmental funding.

Besides implant journals, periodontology and oral and maxillofacial surgery journals have also been major publishing grounds for implant manuscripts, as demonstrated previously by the H-classics method [9]. Consistent to our results, it was reported that *Journal of Clinical Periodontology* and *Journal of Periodontology* have been publishing many highly cited implant articles [10], and that implantology was the most frequent field of publication in *Journal of Oral and Maxillofacial Surgery* and *International Journal of Oral and Maxillofacial Surgery* [33]. Despite the changes in the dental implant research field, *Clinical Oral Implants Research* has stayed in the mainstream. Regardless of whether the time frame was across the entire half-century period or limited to the last decade, *Clinical Oral Implants Research* was responsible for around one tenth of publications. In 2016, it had the highest Impact Factor, Immediacy Index and Eigenfactor Score. The performances of the dental journals publishing dental implant literature have been relatively consistent over the last decade in terms of Impact Factor, Immediacy Index and Eigenfactor Score. In particular, *Clinical Oral Implants Research, Clinical Implant Dentistry and Related Research* and *Journal of Periodontology* had the best and generally increasing Impact Factor and Immediacy Index, whereas *Clinical Oral Implants Research, Journal of Periodontology* and *Journal of Oral and Maxillofacial Surgery* had the best Eigenfactor Score. These findings are comparable to a previous study that reported the relative consistency of performance indices of the top five and bottom five dental journals [22]. From a recent citation analysis of the implant literature [14], papers dealing with peri-implantitis and implant survival / success / failure had higher averaged citation count than papers dealing with other topics. As implant dentistry is becoming more popular and readily available to patients, we expect these journals would publish more papers related to these hot topics and continue to have an increasing Impact Factor in the near future.

The scientific value or academic impact of the research findings or ideas reported from an article or review will eventually depend on its usage. With regards to dental implant research, findings should ultimately inform or transform clinical practice instead of staying merely as a piece of scientific publication. However, most of the key bibliometric indices are based on citation analysis of the journals instead of the individual articles or reviews. Moreover, citations themselves may not accurately reflect the academic merit earned by the cited publications. For instance, a paper could be cited to highlight its flaws [34]. Researchers may read an article or review, discuss it with colleagues, cite it, teach students based on its findings, or incorporate the findings into their evidence-based practice of dentistry. However, the current performance indices of the journals are unable to determine which actions readers have taken after reading the articles or reviews.

There are so-called altmetrics that track and evaluate the impact of articles apart from citation count; for instance, by recording the number of mentions in Twitter, Facebook, Wikipedia, news blogs, etc. [35–38] Similar to citation count, these altmetrics are also tracked by different companies, such as Altmetric and PlumX, which have different counts and give different weights to the individual components to be tracked. Several studies have concluded that the altmetrics data cannot correlate well with the citation count data and are concentrated on recent publications, meaning that the publications published before the introduction of the altmetrics often receive zero or very low score of altmetrics count [35–38].

It should be noted that this study was limited to analyses of publication trend as well as bibliometric data of dental implant articles and reviews without investigating the publication contents. The results from this study should be interpreted together with those from other studies that investigated the types of clinical information contained in dental implant publications [17], publication bias of implant journals [15, 16], the source of funding and internationalization of dental implant journals [19], and the trend of surgical and prosthetic topics concerning dental implantology [11]. From previous studies it seems that the research topics gaining popularity in recent years have been immediate loading, platform switching, lateral sinus grafting, flapless implant surgery and guided implant surgery [11]. Meanwhile, the all-time most cited dental implant articles were mainly dealing with implant success/survival, peri-implant tissue healing and health, guided bone regeneration and biomechanical topics [10, 39]. Implant outcome and peri-implantitis were keywords with increased citations since 2014 [14]. All these findings have suggested that the clinical research of dental implant has been popular and may readily be translated to clinical practice.

As for future perspectives, previous studies have suggested that most of the dental implant publications reported positive significant results [15, 16]; future studies can also consider evaluating if the dental implant journals are willing to publish replication studies or not. As in the fields of neuroscience [40] and psychology [41] journals usually do not explicitly welcome replication studies in their aims and scope and instructions to authors, this may be explored in dental implant field to help understand the publication bias issue. Together, these findings should be able to give the readers a better understanding and more comprehensive picture of the dental implant literature.

4. Conclusion

The current book chapter has summarized the results from a bibliometric study on dental implant literature over the last 50 years. Precisely, the publication data extracted from Web of

Science online database was broken down and analyzed according to the background of the articles and reviews in terms of authors, countries/territories, affiliations and journals. The number of dental implant publications has grown steadily since the 1990s, with the United States being the most productive country and Europe being the predominant continent in terms of publishing. Four of the five journals with the highest numbers of dental implant publications were dedicated to dental implant researches. *Clinical Oral Implants Research* accounted for 11% of total publications. It was also the best performing journal within this research field in 2014, topping the most productive journals with dental implant publications in terms of Impact Factor, Immediacy Index and Eigenfactor Score. The distribution of publications followed Price's law among the authors but had more journals publishing the first one-third of all papers than predicted by Bradford's law.

Acknowledgements

The work described in this paper was partially supported by a grant from the Research Grants Council of the Hong Kong Special Administrative Region, China (HKU 772110 M).

Conflict of interest

The authors declare no conflict of interest.

Author details

Andy Wai Kan Yeung[1]* and Wai Keung Leung[2]

*Address all correspondence to: ndyeung@hku.hk

1 Oral and Maxillofacial Radiology, Applied Oral Sciences, Faculty of Dentistry, The University of Hong Kong, Hong Kong, China

2 Periodontology, Faculty of Dentistry, The University of Hong Kong, Hong Kong, China

References

[1] De Bruyn H, Collaert B, Lindén U, Björn A. Patient's opinion and treatment outcome of fixed rehabilitation on Branemark implants. A 3-year follow-up study in private dental practices. Clinical Oral Implants Research. 1997;**8**(4):265-271

[2] Pjetursson BE, Karoussis I, Bürgin W, Brägger U, Lang NP. Patients' satisfaction following implant therapy. Clinical Oral Implants Research. 2005;**16**(2):185-193

[3] Zitzmann NU, Scherrer SS, Weiger R, Lang NP, Walter C. Preferences of dental care providers in maintaining compromised teeth in relation to their professional status: Implants instead of periodontally involved maxillary molars? Clinical Oral Implants Research. 2011;**22**(2):143-150

[4] Gapski R, Wang HL, Mascarenhas P, Lang NP. Critical review of immediate implant loading. Clinical Oral Implants Research. 2003;**14**(5):515-527

[5] Jung RE, Pjetursson BE, Glauser R, Zembic A, Zwahlen M, Lang NP. A systematic review of the 5-year survival and complication rates of implant-supported single crowns. Clinical Oral Implants Research. 2008;**19**(2):119-130

[6] Lang NP, Pjetursson BE, Tan K, Brägger U, Egger M, Zwahlen M. A systematic review of the survival and complication rates of fixed partial dentures (FPDs) after an observation period of at least 5 years. Clinical Oral Implants Research. 2004;**15**(6):643-653

[7] Lang NP, Pun L, Lau KY, Li KY, Wong M. A systematic review on survival and success rates of implants placed immediately into fresh extraction sockets after at least 1 year. Clinical Oral Implants Research. 2012;**23**(s5):39-66

[8] Chiang HS, Huang RY, Weng PW, Mau LP, Tsai YWC, Chung MP, et al. Prominence of scientific publications toward peri-implant complications in implantology: A bibliometric analysis using the H-classics method. Journal of Oral Rehabilitation. 2018;**45**:240-249

[9] De la Flor-Martínez M, Galindo-Moreno P, Sánchez-Fernández E, Piattelli A, Cobo MJ, Herrera-Viedma E. H-classic: A new method to identify classic articles in implant dentistry, periodontics, and oral surgery. Clinical Oral Implants Research. 2016;**27**(10): 1317-1330

[10] Fardi A, Kodonas K, Lillis T, Veis A. Top-cited articles in implant dentistry. The International Journal of Oral & Maxillofacial Implants. 2017;**32**(3):555-564

[11] Pommer B, Valkova V, Ubaidha Maheen C, Fürhauser L, Rausch-Fan X, Seeman R. Scientific interests of 21st century clinical oral implant research: Topical trend analysis. Clinical Implant Dentistry and Related Research. 2016;**18**(4):850-856

[12] Tarazona B, Vidal-Infer A, Alonso-Arroyo A. Bibliometric analysis of the scientific production in implantology (2009-2013). Clinical Oral Implants Research. 2017;**28**:864-870

[13] Tarazona B, Vidal-Infer A, Tarazona-Alvarez P, Alonso-Arroyo A. Analysis of scientific production in Spanish implantology. Journal of Clinical and Experimental Dentistry. 2017;**9**(5):e703-ee11

[14] Yeung AWK, Leung WK. Citation network analysis of dental implant literature from 2007 to 2016. International Journal of Oral & Maxillofacial Implants. 2018;(accepted)

[15] Yuan JC-C, Shyamsunder N, Adelino Ricardo Barão V, Lee DJ, Sukotjo C. Publication bias in five dental implant journals: An observation from 2005 to 2009. The International Journal of Oral & Maxillofacial Implants. 2011;**26**(5):1024-1032

[16] Papageorgiou SN, Kloukos D, Petridis H, Pandis N. Publication of statistically significant research findings in prosthodontics & implant dentistry in the context of other dental specialties. Journal of Dentistry. 2015;**43**(10):1195-1202

[17] Russo SP, Fiorellini JP, Weber H-P, Niederman R. Benchmarking the dental implant evidence on MEDLINE. The International Journal of Oral & Maxillofacial Implants. 2000;**15**(6):792-800

[18] Barão VAR, Shyamsunder N, Yuan JC-C, Lee DJ, Assunção WG, Sukotjo C. Authorship, collaboration, and funding trends in implantology literature: Analysis of five journals from 2005 to 2009. Implant Dentistry. 2011;**20**(1):68-75

[19] Barão VAR, Shyamsunder N, Yuan JCC, Knoernschild KL, Assunção WG, Sukotjo C. Trends in funding, internationalization, and types of study for original articles published in five implant-related journals between 2005 and 2009. The International Journal of Oral & Maxillofacial Implants. 2012;**27**(1):69-76

[20] Vere J, Joshi R. Quality assessment of prospective case series of dental implant surgery and prosthodontics published between 2004 and 2008: A systematic review. The International Journal of Oral & Maxillofacial Implants. 2012;**27**(4):865-876

[21] Faggion C, Liu J, Huda F, Atieh M. Assessment of the quality of reporting in abstracts of systematic reviews with meta-analyses in periodontology and implant dentistry. Journal of Periodontal Research. 2014;**49**(2):137-142

[22] Jayaratne YSN, Zwahlen RA. The evolution of dental journals from 2003 to 2012: A bibliometric analysis. PLoS One. 2015;**10**(3):e0119503

[23] López-Abente G, Muñoz-Tinoco C. Time trends in the impact factor of public health journals. BMC Public Health. 2005;**5**(1):1

[24] Rosenkrantz AB, Ayoola A. The impact factor of radiological journals: Associations with journal content and other characteristics over a recent 12-year period. Academic Radiology. 2016;**23**(6):661-668. DOI: 10.1016/j.acra.2015.12.026

[25] Chew M, Villanueva EV, Van Der Weyden MB. Life and times of the impact factor: Retrospective analysis of trends for seven medical journals (1994-2005) and their Editors' views. Journal of the Royal Society of Medicine. 2007;**100**(3):142-150

[26] van Eck NJ, Waltman L, van Raan AF, Klautz RJ, Peul WC. Citation analysis may severely underestimate the impact of clinical research as compared to basic research. PLoS One. 2013;**8**(4):e62395

[27] Yeung AWK. Bibliometric study on functional magnetic resonance imaging literature (1995-2017) concerning chemosensory perception. Chemosensory Perception. 2018; [Epub ahead of print]. DOI: 10.1007/s12078-018-9243-0

[28] Yeung AWK, Goto TK, Leung WK. A bibliometric review of research trends in neuroimaging. Current Science. 2017;**112**(4):725-734. DOI: 10.18520/cs/v112/i04/725-734

[29] Yeung AWK, Goto TK, Leung WK. The changing landscape of neuroscience research, 2006-2015: A bibliometric study. Frontiers in Neuroscience. 2017;**11**:120

[30] Yeung AWK, Goto TK, Leung WK. At the leading front of neuroscience: A bibliometric study of the 100 most-cited articles. Frontiers in Human Neuroscience. 2017;**11**:363

[31] Nicholls PT. Price's square root law: Empirical validity and relation to Lotka's law. Information Processing and Management. 1988;**24**(4):469-477

[32] Chen Y-S, Leimkuhler FF. A relationship between Lotka's law, Bradford's law, and Zipf's law. Journal of the American Society for Information Science. 1986;**37**(5):307

[33] Aslam-Pervez N, Lubek JE. Most cited publications in oral and maxillofacial surgery: A bibliometric analysis. Oral and Maxillofacial Surgery. 2018;**22**(1):25-37

[34] White HD. Citation analysis and discourse analysis revisited. Applied Linguistics. 2004;**25**(1):89-116

[35] Costas R, Zahedi Z, Wouters P. Do "altmetrics" correlate with citations? Extensive comparison of altmetric indicators with citations from a multidisciplinary perspective. Journal of the Association for Information Science and Technology. 2015;**66**(10):2003-2019

[36] Priem J, Groth P, Taraborelli D. The altmetrics collection. PLoS One. 2012;**7**(11):e48753

[37] Thelwall M, Haustein S, Larivière V, Sugimoto CR. Do altmetrics work? Twitter and ten other social web services. PLoS One. 2013;**8**(5):e64841

[38] Zahedi Z, Costas R, Wouters P. How well developed are altmetrics? A cross-disciplinary analysis of the presence of 'alternative metrics' in scientific publications. Scientometrics. 2014;**101**(2):1491-1513

[39] Antonio Alarcón M, Esparza D, Montoya C, Monje A, Faggion CM Jr. The 300 most-cited articles in implant dentistry. The International Journal of Oral & Maxillofacial Implants. 2017;**32**(1):e8-e22

[40] Yeung AWK. Do neuroscience journals accept replications? A survey of literature. Frontiers in Human Neuroscience. 2017;**11**:468

[41] Martin G, Clarke RM. Are psychology journals anti-replication? A snapshot of editorial practices. Frontiers in Psychology. 2017;**8**:523

Section 2

Updates on Grafting and Surgical Techniques of Implant Fixture Management

Chapter 2

Immediate Implantation at Fresh Extraction Sockets

Belir Atalay

Additional information is available at the end of the chapter

http://dx.doi.org/10.5772/intechopen.78969

Abstract

The term 'osseointegration' was first defined by Branemark in 1952. Osseointegration means direct connection between implant surface and live bone cells. At the beginning, the original protocol for installation of the dental implants was 6–8 months after extraction. After installation of the implant, waiting period for osseointegration time was 6 months for upper jaw and 3 months for the lower jaw. In 1990s, implant placement was mostly performed in 100% healed bone tissue. Today this approach has lost its dominance due to the evolution of the implant shape and surface features. Various studies show that immediate implantation has a 90–100% success in survival rate. However, primary stability of the implant at the fresh extraction socket still has a priority. Particularly after extraction of single root teeth implant, installation into the fresh extraction socket by filling the gap with graft materials come into prominence. Many types of graft materials can be used with or without plasma-rich materials like Plasma Rich Fibrin (PRF). Recent studies have shown that these kind of materials enhance the osteogenic regeneration. Immediate implantation proved that it reduces the total treatment time, prevents the loss of gummy tissues and gains esthetic success.

Keywords: immediate implant, bone graft, bone healing, fresh extraction socket, tooth extraction, osseointegration

1. Introduction

Amler describes the healing process into five stages. In the first stage after tooth extraction, hemorrhage and coagulum formation occurs. In the second stage, resorption of the coagulum and granulation formation over the clot occurs after 5 days period. In the third stage, new form of connective tissue begins to form over granulation tissue with early angiogenesis and this occurs over 14–16 days. At the fourth stage, apparently osteoid tissue begins to identify and to fill the whole socket with bone takes about 6 weeks. At the last stage, complete epithelial closure of the socket occurs in almost 25 days and the extraction socket is fulfilled with bone approximately in 16 weeks [1]. The highest osteoblastic activity occurs between 4 and 6 weeks and after 8th week, this process begins to slow down [2]. This progress has been found by histologic examination of human extraction socket biopsies and animal histologic materials [3–5].

After extraction, there will be a resorption period at the same time with the healing process. It is a physiological mechanism and in the first year after extraction its effect is higher than the following years. There are many studies that measure the resorption of the alveolar bone quantity after tooth extraction. Different methods were used for this purpose, direct measurement by the time of implant surgery [6–9]. Study cast measurement, cephalometric measurements and subtraction radiography methods were also used for this purpose [6, 7, 10–13].

During post-extraction period in the first year, the alveolar bone loss is calculated about 4 mm in bone height and 25% loss in total volume [12]. At the same study, scientists report that 40–60% of bone loss occurs in 3 years after tooth extraction. Christensen et al. reported that in long-term period, the resorption at the extraction site was 0.5–1%. These physiological changes can potentially be seen in every patient. Approximately 6 mm bone resorption is identified over 6–12 months and 50% of this bone resorption is horizontal alveolar ridge reduction [10, 14]. The vertical ridge loss was measured as 2–4 mm by researchers. And this can be more than 4 mm. when multiple extractions performed [14, 15]. After 6 months post extraction, approximately 50% of the vertical resorption has been reported [6, 7]. Both vertical and horizontal bone resorption over a 12 month period occurred simultaneously together. Most of this process occurs in the first 3 months after the extraction. After 12 months, crestal bone levels at the tooth surfaces neighbor to the extracted tooth remained almost same with the amount of 0.1 mm bone loss. The newly formed bone at the extraction socket cannot reach the bone level of the neighbor teeth [11, 16].

There are many factors which may affect these resorption process such as systemic factors, patient habits and general health conditions, local extraction trauma, periodontitis, socket wall conditions, number of extracted adjacent teeth, differences between mouth and dental arches, the biotype of the soft tissues and the type of temporary prosthesis if applied [16]. Besides those factors, the pattern and rate of resorption may be changed if traumatic extraction, pathologic processes or occlusal trauma have damaged one or more bony walls of the socket [17]. There is still insufficient scientific studies about the differences between rates and healing patterns of damaged and intact sockets [16].

Literature suggested guideline for implantation was waiting for alveolar ridge remodeling and healing for 3 months after tooth extraction. And 3–6 months stress free submerged healing without loading was needed for osseointegration [18–20]. At the beginning in 1952, the original Branemark protocol for installation of implants was minimum 6 months waiting-healing period of extraction sockets [21, 22]. Generally the two stage approach was applied; first surgery implant placement and after 3–6 months of submerged healing period, the second surgery applied to open the implant into the mouth. It took approximately 1 year for the final implant supported restoration [12, 23]. This extended treatment time generally necessitate a removable prosthesis enhance cost of the treatment and inconvenience at the patients.

Recently against earlier protocols, need for a faster and more affordable treatment type has gain necessity. There has been increasing interest in immediate implantation [24]. There are several classifications till 1990 to describe the timing of implantation. Mayfield discussed the procedure based on timing after tooth extraction. The terms immediate, delayed and late are used to describe time intervals of 0 weeks, 6–10 weeks and 6 months or more after tooth extraction [25]. Wilson and Weber make a classification based on soft tissue healing but without time intervals [26]. The terms immediate, recent, delayed and mature are used to describe the timing of implantation in relation to soft tissue healing [26]. Hammerle et al. proposed a new one in 2004 that was based on soft and hard tissue healing a classification of four categories (Type1–4). Type I describes immediate implantation after tooth extraction at the same day. Type II describes implantation after complete soft tissue healing typically 4–8 weeks after extraction. Type III was implantation after clinical and/or radiographic bone fill of the extraction socket typically 12–16 weeks after extraction. And Type IV describes the implantation after complete bone fill of the socket means typically more than 16 weeks after extraction [27].

Today well accepted terminology of immediate implantation includes immediate, early and late placement of implants at the post-extraction sockets [28, 29]. Immediate implant placement means implantation at the same time instantly after extraction into the extraction socket. Early placement is 2–4 week delayed implantation after extraction and allowing soft tissue healing. And delayed approach is the conventional method describes implantation after 4–6 months of waiting for complete healing time [27].

There are many advantages of immediate implantation. With this procedure, there is a reduction in the number of surgeries and shorten total treatment time. Also immediate implantation preserves the bone and soft tissues at the extraction socket [30–36]. It decreases the morbidity and rehabilitation time associated with crown replacement and increases patient satisfaction with treatment [32, 37, 38]. However, there is a higher risk for implant failure, unpredictable hard and soft tissue changes and difficulty at primary stabilization [27]. Early placement is also shorten the treatment time but requires an extra surgical procedure and waiting for 2–4 weeks post-extraction allows soft tissue healing. Conventional delayed implantation takes the longest treatment time, requires extra surgical intervention and bone resorption during healing, however, that procedure have less implant failure risk [27, 39]. The short-term survival rate of the methods seems similar between each other. However, there is still little data on the success rates [27].

2. Immediate implantation indications and contraindications

For immediate implantation, it is better to provide ideal clinical conditions. The evaluation of gingival type, facial bone wall, level of smile line, hard and soft tissue levels must be evaluated [40, 41]. When full intact of facial bone with thick phenotype of gingival tissue represents there is a very low risk of gingival recession at the neck of the implant prosthesis. If implant placement is done in patients with a thin biotype, there will be a high risk of thread exposion. Because thin gingival biotype has higher frequency for gingival recession when compared with thick biotypes. As a result, immediate implantation at the areas with thin tissue biotypes is often not recommended [42, 43]. There must be no an acute or purulent infection at the extraction socket or close to the socket. When chronic infection presents at the extracted tooth area, it can be a concern to place an immediate implant, although not all authors agree for that. Currently, it is agreed that immediate implantation can be performed at the same time with the extraction of periapical lesion sites as long as the infection is removed totally and implant primary stability achieved [27]. Periodontal biotype affects periodontal tissue dimensions and esthetic outcomes [40]. It should be sufficient bony walls at the apical and palatal sites of the socket though implant need to be primarily stabilized and the 3D positioning should be acceptable [44]. For predictable outcome of immediately, replaced single tooth implant success, Kois addresses five diagnostic factors. These are:

1. Tooth position relatively with free gingiva margin,
2. Biotype of the periodontium,
3. Form of the periodontium,
4. Condition of the crestal bone before extraction,
5. Tooth shape.

These factors should be analyzed carefully before immediate implant placement [41]. When there is an option for flapless surgery, it is the ideal circumstance compared with open, flap procedure. With flapless surgery, there will be less recession of the peri-implanter area. Flapless immediate implant placement offers least morbidity for the patients. Although it might seem to be a simple surgery, it is considered as a complex one [44]. It is not easy to prepare a new implant socket at the same extraction socket. Procedure needs a skilled surgeon with experience. New implant socket must be prepared more palatally and avoid any palatal or buccal perforation. To avoid any perforation risks or malposition of implant, guided surgery can be performed or the surgeon should be experienced for the procedure. Corono-apically, the implant should be placed deep inside the extraction socket. The distance between implant shoulder and mid-facial bone crest should be 0.5–1 mm [45]. In some cases, this amount reaches up to 2 mm. This approach avoids worse esthetic outcomes according to the bone resorption. Also distance between implant shoulder and internal surface of the facial bone wall should be at least 2 mm [46]. That gap provides a space for the formation of a blood clot. And from that clot, provisional connective tissue matrix is organized. This change in time to the newly formed woven bone [44]. This gap can be filled with appropriate bone grafts and it is recommended by many researchers and clinicians. Bone grafts reduce the amount of post-surgical buccal bone resorption [47].

To generalize indications, immediate implantation should be performed at systemically healthy patients without acute infection areas and who has adequate hard and soft tissues with intact facial plate and thick tissue biotype. The absolute contraindications are patients with complicated systemic disease, history of iv bisphosphonates usage, uncontrolled periodontal disease, absence of intact labial bone and presence of acute infection. Heavy smokers and maxillary sinus involvements are relative contraindications [27].

3. Surgical procedure

For achieving successful long-term results with immediate implant placement at the fresh extraction sockets, there are some essential rules to obey. In each patient, periapical and panaromic X-rays and computerized tomography scans should be obtained if necessary. If there is no contraindication for the patients administration of local anesthesia, 2% Articaine HCl with 1:100,000 epinephrine was performed. No incisions should be made and no flaps should be reflected unless necessary. At the beginning, an atraumatic tooth extraction is important. Sharp and thin devices like periotomes may be better to use subcrestally when dissecting the fibers. Tooth should be elevated with minimal trauma to the alveolus and rotational movement is better to achieve. Surgeon should avoid to damage the buccal plate and for that it is important to avoid bucco-lingual movement [48]. When the extraction performed at the molar area sometimes endodontically treated roots, multiple roots and curved roots can make the extraction more challenging. Mostly root fracturing can happen. Leaving root tips that can leave the surgeon in medico legal jeopardy to avoid this, it is too important for the surgeon not to leave any root particles in the extraction socket. It is better to use diamond burrs for cutting roots coronally. If there is chronic infection at the socket area, all residual infected remnants must be removed properly. After curettage, the area intrabone marrow penetration with round burrs and curretes can stimulate bleeding and this allows bone fill with maximum amounts [27]. Implant must be placed into enough natural bone with enough primary stability apically or laterally in an ideal three-dimensional position at the extraction socket. Placement of the implant, 3–5 mm apically into the socket or using wide diameter implants increase primary stability. Also placing the implant 2–3 mm below cement-enamel junction of adjacent tooth will provide a better outcome [30, 49, 50].

To prevent buccal plate damage, Yalcin et al. developed an extraction technique in 2009. In this technique in order not to traumatize the surrounding bone during elevation, implant drills were placed in root canals to thin out the root walls giving enough space to extract tooth without applying much more force. It is better to use thin and sharp drills at the beginning. The diameter of the drills should be increased after first sharp drill. Recommended diameter after first drill is 2 mm pilot drill and afterwards it can be increased according to the implant system and the diameter of the tooth. Before final drilling, it is better to extract thin walls of the root from the extraction socket. Preparing the implant site using drills as palatally as possible is recommended. When the socket is ready for implant placement, a periodontal probe should use to explore and estimate the integrity of the alveolar bone. Periapical radiographs can be taken to confirm the total removal of the root remnants. To maintain primary stability, it is better to place long and wide implants as much as possible. After placing the implant, filling the gap between implant and buccal bone with bone graft is recommended [51]. (**Figures 1–13**) There are many different graft types that used in oral and maxillofacial surgery. The gold standard material for grafting procedure is autogenous graft. Preparing the extraction socket for immediate implantation may provide to collect some autogenous bone graft material. Besides this there are many different graft types, for healing process there is no difference between graft types was found that filled the gap around immediately placed implants. Scientific data about this topic assumes the gold standard for grafting was autogenous

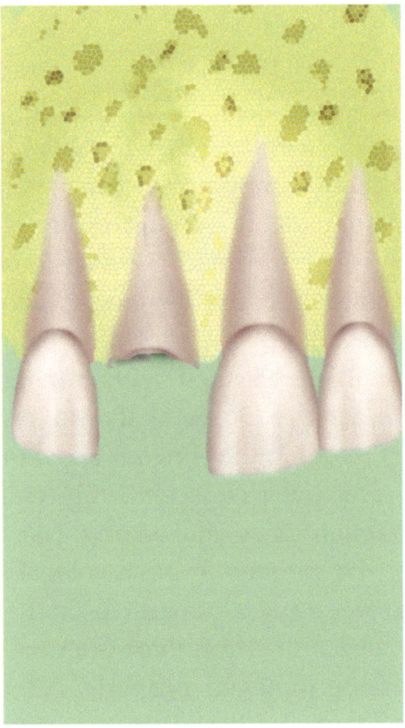

Figure 1. Schematic view of a broken tooth deep in the socket.

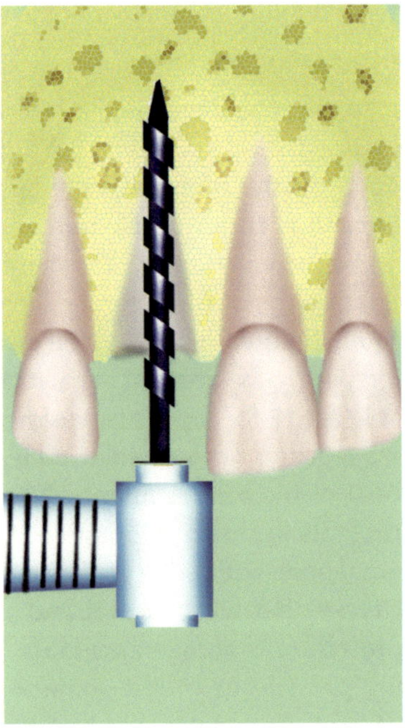

Figure 2. Thinning the walls of the root with a thin and sharp pilot drill. The first drill should move through the root approximately 3–10 mm in depth.

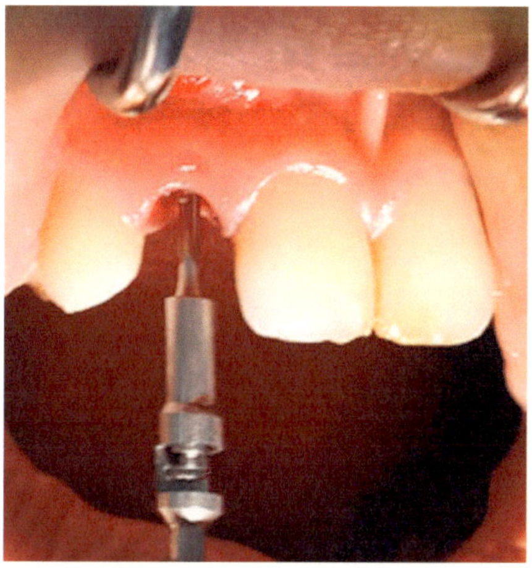

Figure 3. Drilling the root with a 2 mm sharp first drill.

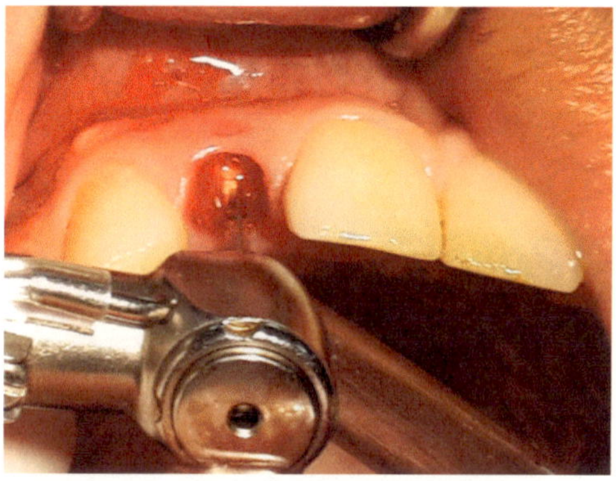

Figure 4. Drilling starts at the center of the root moves apically to palatally.

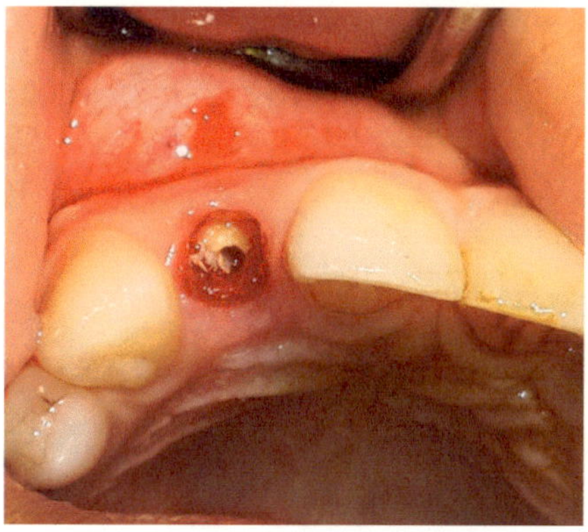

Figure 5. First 2 mm drill compose a cavity at the center of the root.

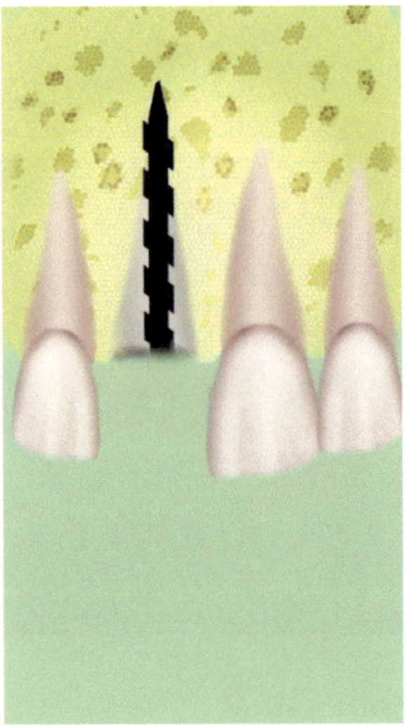

Figure 6. After first drill, a schematic view of the root remnants.

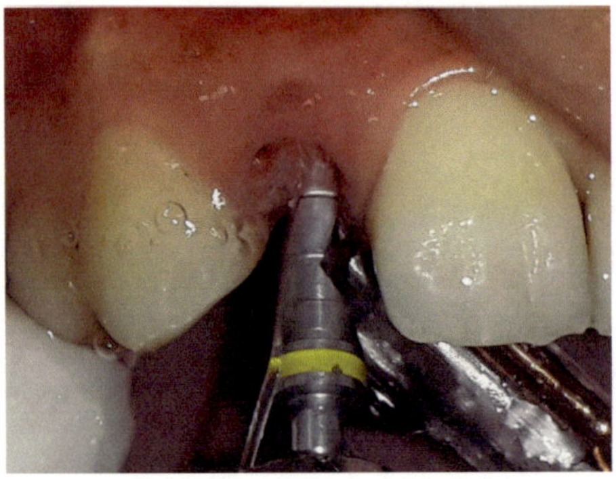

Figure 7. Thinning the walls of the root with thicker 2.2, 3.5 mm drill/drills that depend on the implant system.

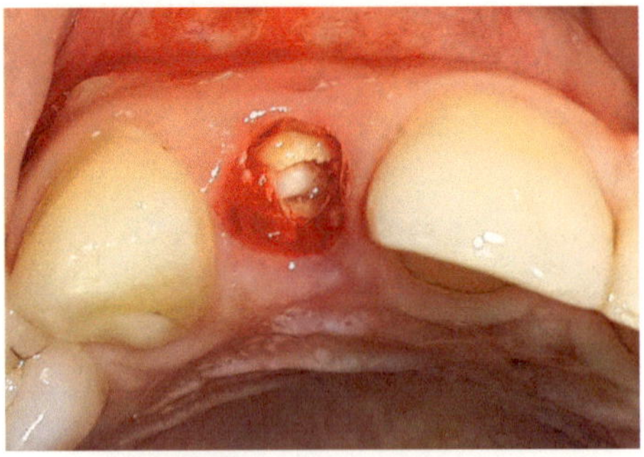

Figure 8. Occlusal view of root remnants after drilling.

http://dx.doi.org/10.5772/intechopen.78969

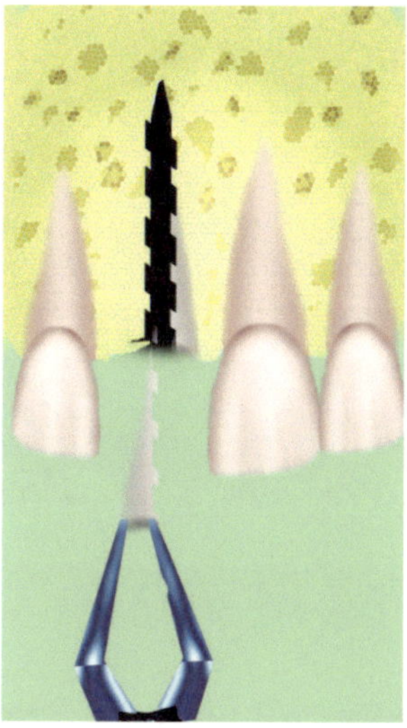

Figure 9. Root remnants should be separated from the alveolar bone with the help of a sharp device like periotome. Later separation of remnants removed from the socket by root forceps. Schematic view of removing root remnants before placing implant from the extraction socket.

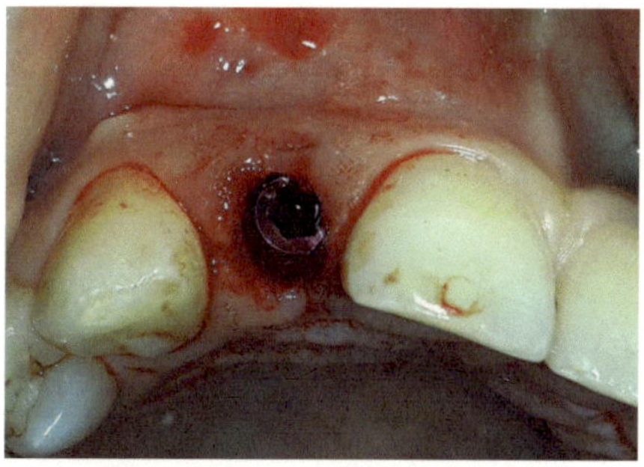

Figure 10. Replacing the implant to the cavity by handpiece or manual device.

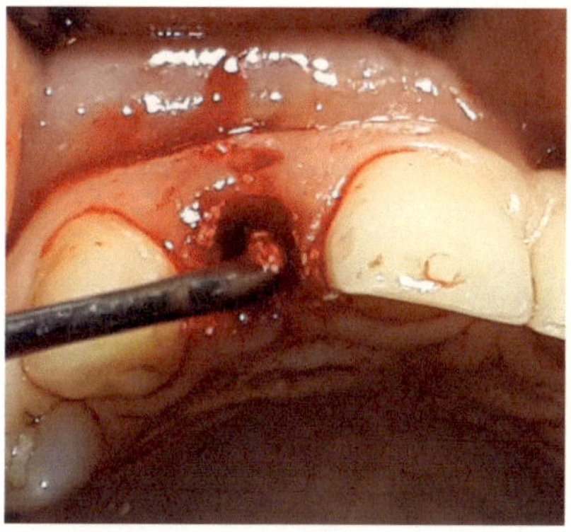

Figure 11. Filling the gap between implant and buccal bone with grafting material. It is important to fill the gap with graft material to prevent soft tissue migration.

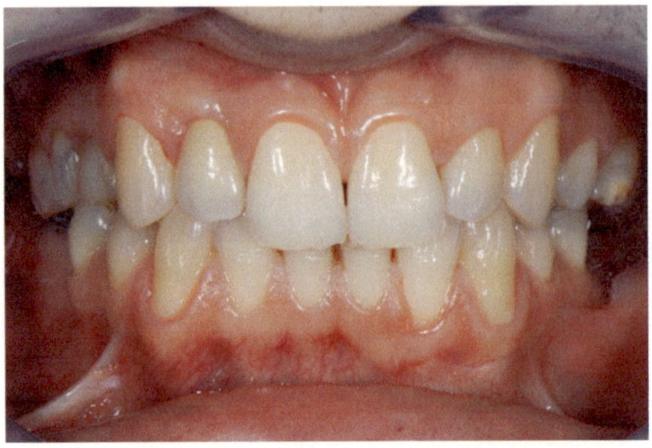

Figure 12. Final prosthesis.

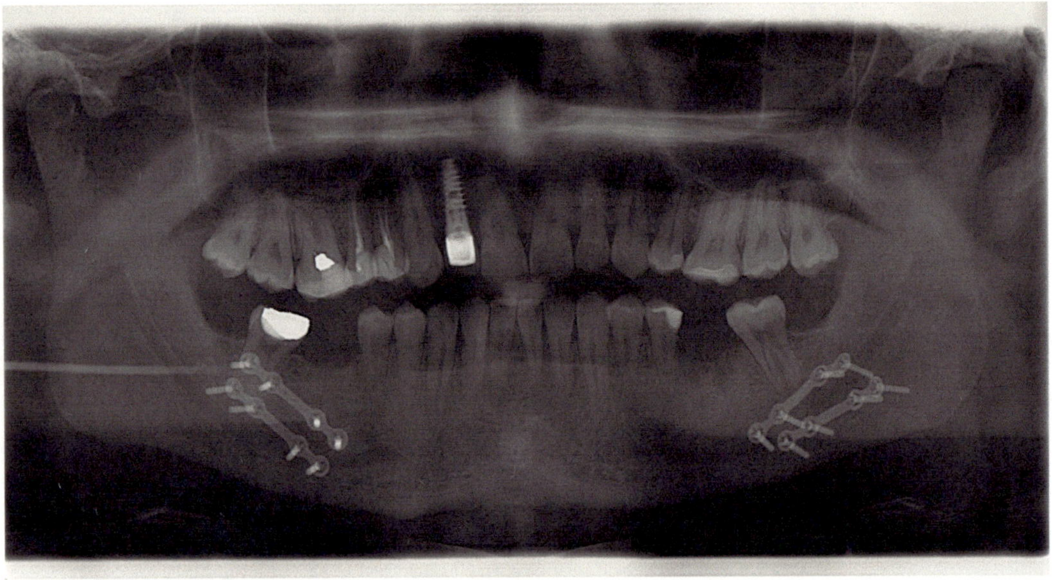

Figure 13. Final X-ray.

grafting. But resorption tendency for autogenous graft material was found high in this kind of graft material. In clinical practice, the need for second surgery area for autogenous graft collection makes the procedure more complicated, although any synthetic graft material can be preferred for grafting procedure.

Surgical area was closed using 4-0 silk, rapid vicryl or 5-0 monofilament resorbable sutures as preferred by the surgeon. Regular medicine included 1 g amoxicillin, non-steroidal analgesics and chlorhexidine gluconate mouth rinse twice a day for 5 days were prescribed to the patients. Penicillin-sensitive patients were prescribed azithromycin or clarithromycin. When using particulated bone grafting materials, antibiotics may prevent possible infection. Systemic antibiotics were used generally in accordance with surgery, whether in conjuction with immediate, early, delayed or late implantation. However, the effect of antibiotic usage on outcome is still unknown [52–59].

Waiting for healing time for osseointegration of the implants varies between 6 weeks for mandible and 8 weeks for maxilla to 12 weeks post-surgery depending on the system of the implant. Time can be extended 4–6 months post surgically. After the end of the waiting time, a re-entry is necessary for the implant if immediate temporary crown was not applied. Generally, 1 week of waiting for the gingival healing is enough for impression. The final crown can be applied either cemented or screw retained and can be loaded into function.

4. Immediate implant placement at maxillary molars

Most delay reason for implantation at the maxillary molar area is the proximity to the maxillary sinus floor. Amount of bone left on the floor of the maxillary sinus after tooth extraction defined the treatment plan. Distance between the sinus floor and the root apex should be min 3 mm for the best clinical outcome. Also the thickness between roots affects the primary stability at the same area. When tooth has deep decays or crown fractures, separating the roots and moving out them gently is recommended. Best place to prepare implant cavity is the bone center of three roots. If there is enough bone thickness and height for drilling, widest implant in diameter is recommended. After placing the implant, gaps around the implant and the bone border should be filled with bone graft substitutes. With that approach after achieving implant stability, the success rate is approximately 95–97% [60]. When drilling if the height of the bone is not sufficient, bone condensing with internal sinus lift through the maxillary sinus recommended. If there is inadequate bone for stabilizing the implant or the position of the implant does not allow a crown in an ideal position, immediate implantation can be canceled. After 3–4 months, implant can be placed with additional open or internal sinus lift at that time. Perforation of the sinus membrane can be seen but if the bone height is 4 mm or more, implant can be placed normally.

5. Immediate implant placement at mandibular molars

The most avoided procedure for clinicians is immediate implantation at mandibular molar area. This is because of presence of nervus alveolaris inferior and linea obliqua interna. Inter radicular septum bone is highly recommended place for replacing the implant. To avoid traumatizing that area extraction should be done atraumatically. Sometimes it is advisable to separate the crown from the roots and the roots from each other. Using sharp devices like periotomes for losing periodontal sharpey fibers should ease the moving of the roots. The height of the bone can change after the extraction. To avoid mandibular nerve injury, intraoperative X-rays can be done during preparation of the implant gap. After every drill, a depth gauge can be placed at the implant gap and with an X-ray it can measure distance to the mandibular canal. After every drill, consecutive depth gauges in different diameters should be placed at the implant gap to determine the amount of bone that holds the implant buccolingually and mesiodistally. Also that may provide not to perforate the lingual cortex. After installing the implant, there can be gaps near the mesial and distal implants. These gaps should be filled with bone graft substitutes. There are some complications that would inhibit immediate implantation at the mandibular molar area. Sometimes, there is inability to remove all infected material from the socket area. It is difficult to place implant in a proper position. To gain primary stabilization can be difficult. Mandibular nerve damage can be happen due to much drilling through the mandibular nerve canal. In case of unfavorable conditions, then a two stage procedure should be performed [60].

6. Complication treatments

Like sinus membrane perforation or nervus alveolaris inferior damage, it is better to wait and see. Sinus membrane heals about 4–8 weeks. At same time with implantation, patients prescribed routine antibiotics and non-steroid anti-inflammatory drugs. Additional nasal pump spray of oxymetazoline HCl was given for 5 days, three times a day for twice pump for each nostril. When nerve damage occurs, it takes quite a lot time for healing. Healing depends on the degree of nerve damage. At the beginning after surgery if it happens, implant should be removed or implant not inserted with dexamethasone can be added to their routine prescription. During surgery, when implants cannot be placed in a proper position, it is better to take it out and drill the cavity for an ideal position and install the implant in a proper position if possible. When there is not enough bone for that, delaying implantation and GBR procedure should be performed. After 3–6 months, delayed implantation protocol is recommended. If implant integrates in a poor position, explantation is indicated [60]. Explantation usually performed with trephine drills fit for implant. It is so important that removing the osseointegrated implant with a trephine drill under serum physiologic irrigation must be done properly to avoid heating bone tissue. Explantation should be done under saline irrigation and without too much pressure. After removal, GBR procedures can be performed with or without soft tissue augmentation. Delayed implantation after 3–6 months can be done. To prevent malposition, surgical guide can be used for ideal positioning.

7. Discussion

Immediate implant placement can be challenging due to unpredictable soft and hard tissue healing. Araujo et al. studied the dimensional changes of alveolar bone after immediate implant placement and buccal bone resorption was noted [61]. However, many other studies found the amount of resorption reduced both delayed and immediate approach resulted in statistically significant reduction [61, 62]. Gher ME et al. reported that significantly better bone fill and less crestal bone resorption at immediate implantation sites treated with demineralized freeze-dried bone combination with non-resorbable barrier membrane [42]. For observing about crestal bone loss for immediately replaced implants, it was very hard to estimate the outcome. In two papers such data showed that after 1 and 5 years, 12 and 18% of the implants has a loss of more than 2 mm of crestal bone loss [42, 63, 64].

For about soft tissue complications, only a prospective study and one retrospective study reported frequency distributions of probing depths around immediately placed implants. After 6 years of immediately placed implants with pockets greater than 4 mm is about 20%. Bianchi et al. reported that pockets greater than 3 mm reached 50% [42, 63, 65]. According to some authors there can be serious gingival recessions that resulted thread exposure with immediate implantation, even though the incidence was not so much [30, 64, 66–69].

Quiryen et al. reflected that total incidence of implant loss after immediate placement was 4–5%. The incidence was greater when immediate placement and immediate loading combined together especially for minimally rough implant surfaces [63].

There is lack of evidence regarding the effect of apical pathology on the success and survival of immediate placed implants. Some studies showed that survival rate of immediately placed implants placed after extraction of tooth with combined endo-perio problems, root fractures and perforations are similar to that of implants placed in healed area [16, 70, 71].

8. Conclusion

Immediate implant placement approach has been known and applied since 1970s and has an increasing attraction. Today the procedure has evident increasing success. Case selection is critical, before like any other surgical approach, a thorough and detailed systemic medical anamnesis and habit history should be obtained. Patient compliance and expectations should determined. Patients who have no systemic problems and healing problems, compliant, thick biotype of soft and bone tissue have the least risk for any complication. Atraumatic extraction of the tooth with preserving the socket bone and papillae means flapless approach has effects outcome success. Also placing the implant in an ideal three-dimensional position is important. When necessary, guided bone regeneration and soft tissue grafting techniques should be well known and applied by the surgeon.

Acknowledgements

Special thanks to Prof Dr. Yusuf Emes for creating figures by drawing.

Conflict of interest

This chapter has no any 'conflict of interest'.

Author details

Belir Atalay

Address all correspondence to: batalay@istanbul.edu.tr

Department of Oral and Maxillofacial Surgery, Istanbul University School of Dentistry, Istanbul, Turkey

References

[1] Amler MH. The time sequence of tissue regeneration in human extraction wounds. Oral Surgery, Oral Medicine, and Oral Pathology. 1969;**27**(3):309-318

[2] Evian CI, Rosenberg ES, Coslet JG, Corn H. The osteogenic activity of bone removed from healing extraction sockets in humans. Journal of Periodontology. 1982;**53**(2):81-85

[3] Huebsch RF, Hansen LS. A histopathologic study of extraction wounds in dogs. Oral Surgery, Oral Medicine, and Oral Pathology. 1969;**282**:187-196

[4] Ohta Y. Comparative changes in microvasculature and bone during healing of implant and extraction sites. The Journal of Oral Implantology. 1993;**193**:184-189

[5] Bodner L, Dayan D, Rothchild D, Hammel I. Extraction wound healing in desalivated rats. Journal of Oral Pathology & Medicine. 1991;**20**:176-178

[6] Lekovic V, Kenney EB, Weinlaender M, Han T, Klokkevold P, Nedic M, Orsini M. A bone regenerative approach to alveolar ridge maintenance following tooth extraction. Report of 10 cases. Journal of Periodontology. 1997;**686**:563-570

[7] Lekovic V, Camargo PM, Klokkevold PR, Weinlaender M, Kenney EB, Dimitrijevic B, Nedic M. Preservation of bone in extraction sockets using bioabsorbable membranes. Journal of Periodontology. 1998;**69**(9):1044-1049

[8] Camargo PM, Lekovic V, Weinlaender M, Klokkevold PR, Kenney EB, Dimitrijevic B, Nedic M, Jancovic S, Orsini M. Influence of bioactive glass on changes in alveolar process dimensions after exodontia. Oral Surgery, Oral Medicine, Oral Pathology, Oral Radiology. 2000;**905**:581-586

[9] Iasella JM, Greenwell H, Miller RL, Hill M, Drisko C, Bohra AA, Scheetz JP. Ridge preservation with freeze-dried bone allograft and a collagen membrane compared to extraction alone for implant site development: A clinical and histologic study in humans. Journal of Periodontology. 2003;**74**:990-999

[10] Johnson K. A study of the dimensional changes occurring in the maxilla after tooth extraction. Part 1: Normal healing. Australian Dental Journal. 1963;**8**:428-434

[11] Schropp L, Wenzel A, Kostopoulos L, Karring T. Bone healing and soft tissue contour changes following single-tooth extraction: A clinical and radiographic 12-month prospective study. The International Journal of Periodontics & Restorative Dentistry. 2003;**23**:313-323

[12] Carlsson GE, Bergman B, Hedegard B. Changes in contour of the maxillary alveolar process under immediate dentures. A longitudinal clinical and X-ray cephalometric study covering 5 years. Acta Odontologica Scandinavica. 1967;**251**:45-75

[13] Atwood DA, Coy WA. Clinical, cephalometric, and densitometric study of reduction of residual ridges. The Journal of Prosthetic Dentistry. 1971;**26**:280-295

[14] Johnson K. A study of dimensional changes occurring in the maxilla following tooth extraction. Australian Dental Journal. 1969;**14**:241-244

[15] Lam RV. Contour changes of the alveolar processes following extraction. The Journal of Prosthetic Dentistry. 1960;**10**:25-32

[16] Chen ST, Wilson TG Jr, Hammerle CH. Immediate or early placement of implants following tooth extraction: Review of biologic basis, clinical procedures, and outcomes. The International Journal of Oral & Maxillofacial Implants. 2004;**19**(Suppl):12-25. Review

[17] Adriens PA. Preservation of bony sites. In: Lindhe J (editor). Proceedings of the 3rd European Workshop in Periodontology: Implant Dentistry. Berlin: Quintessenz; 1999. pp. 266-280

[18] Adell R, Lekholm U, Rockler B, Branemark PI. A 15-year study of osseointegrated implants in the treatment of the edentulous jaw. International Journal of Oral Surgery. 1981;**10**:387-416

[19] Adell R, Eriksson B, Lekholm U, Branemark PI, Jemt T. Longterm follow-up study of osseointegrated implants in the treatment of totally edentulous jaws. The International Journal of Oral & Maxillofacial Implants. 1990;**5**:347-359

[20] Albrektsson T. A multicenter report on osseointegrated oral implants. The Journal of Prosthetic Dentistry. 1988;**60**:75-84

[21] Branemark PI. Osseointegration and its experimental background. The Journal of Prosthetic Dentistry. 1983;**50**(3):399-410

[22] Branemark PI, Adell R, Breine U, Hansson BO, Lindström J, Ohlsson A. Intra-osseous anchorage of dental prostheses. I. Experimental studies. Scandinavian Journal of Plastic and Reconstructive Surgery. 1969;**3**(2):81-100

[23] Branemark PI, Hansson BO, Adell R, Breine U, Lindström J, Hallen O, Ohman A. Osseointegrated implants in the treatment of the edentulous jaw. Experience from a 10-year period. Scandinavian Journal of Plastic and Reconstructive Surgery. Supplementum. 1977;**16**:1-132

[24] Schulte W, Kleineikenscheidt H, Linder K, Schareyka R. Tübingen immediate implant in clinical studies. Deutsche Zahnarztliche Zeitschrift. 1978;**33**:348-359

[25] Mayfield L. Immediate, delayed, and late submerged and transmucosal implants. In: Proceedings of the 3rd European Workshop on Periodontology: Implant Dentistry; 1999. pp. 520-534

[26] Wilson TG, Weber HP. Classification of and therapy for areas of deficient bony housing prior to dental implant placement. The International Journal of Periodontics & Restorative Dentistry. 1993;**13**:451-459

[27] Koh RU, Rudek I, Wang HL. Immediate implant placement: Positives and negatives. Implant Dentistry. 2010;**19**(2):98-108

[28] Hammerle CH, Araujo MG, Simion M. Evidence-based knowledge on the biology and treatment of extraction sockets. Clinical Oral Implants Research. 2012;**23**(Suppl 5):80-82

[29] Schropp L, Isidor F. Timing of implant placement relative to tooth extraction. Journal of Oral Rehabilitation. 2008;**35**(Suppl I):33-43

[30] Lazzara RM. Immediate implant placement into extraction sites: Surgical and restorative advantages. The International Journal of Periodontics & Restorative Dentistry. 1989;**9**:333-343

[31] Parel SM, Triplett RG. Immediate fixture placement: A treatment planning alternative. The International Journal of Oral & Maxillofacial Implants. 1990;**54**:337-345

[32] Werbitt MJ, Goldenberg PV. The immediate implant: Bone preservation and bone regeneration. The International Journal of Periodontics & Restorative Dentistry. 1992;**12**:207-217

[33] Schultz AJ. Guided tissue regeneration (GTR) of nonsubmerged implants in immediate extraction sites. Practical Periodontics and Aesthetic Dentistry. 1993;**52**:59-65

[34] Shanaman RH. The use of guided tissue regeneration to facilitate ideal prosthetic placement of implants. The International Journal of Periodontics & Restorative Dentistry. 1992; **124**:256-265

[35] Denissen HW, Kalk W, Veldhuis HA, van Waas MA. Anatomic consideration for preventive implantation. The International Journal of Oral & Maxillofacial Implants. 1993;**82**:191-196

[36] Watzek G, Haider R, Mensdorff-Pouilly N, Haas R. Immediate and delayed implantation for complete restoration of the jaw following extraction of all residual teeth: A retrospective study comparing different types of serial immediate implantation. The International Journal of Oral & Maxillofacial Implants. 1995;**105**:561-567

[37] Lindeboom JA, Tjiook Y, Kroon FH. Immediate placement of implants in periapical infected sites: A prospective randomized study in 50 patients. Oral Surgery, Oral Medicine, Oral Pathology, Oral Radiology, and Endodontics. 2006;**101**:705-710

[38] Agliardi E, Panigatti S, Clerico M, Villa C, Malo P. Immediate rehabilitation of the edentulous jaws with full fixed prostheses supported by four implants: Interinm results of a single cohort prospective study. Clinical Oral Implants Research. 2010;**21**:459-465

[39] Esposito M, Grusovin MG, Chew YS, Coulthard P, Worthington HV. Interventions for replacing missing teeth: 1-versus 2- stage implant placement. Cochrane Database of Systematic Reviews. 2009;**3**:CD006698

[40] Kan JY, Rungcharassaeng K, Umezu K, Kois JC. Dimensions of peri-implant mucosa: An evaluation of maxillary anterior single implants in humans. Journal of Periodontology. 2003;**74**:557-562

[41] Kois JC. Predictable single-tooth peri-implant esthetics: Five diagnostic keys. The Compendium of Continuing Education in Dentistry. 2004;**25**:895-896, 898,900 passim; quiz 906-897

[42] Gher ME, Quintero G, Assad D, Monaco E, Richardsson AC. Bone grafting and guided bone regeneration for immediate dental implants in humans. Journal of Periodontology. 1994;**65**:881-891

[43] Boticelli D, Berglundh T, Lindhe J. Hard tissue alterations following immediate implant placement in extraction sites. Journal of Clinical Periodontology. 2004;**31**:820-828

[44] Buser D, Chappuis V, Belser UC, Chen S. Implant placement post extraction in esthetic single tooth sites: When immediate, when early, when late? Periodontology 2000. 2017;**73**: 84-102

[45] Chen ST, Darby I. The relationship between facial bone wall defects and dimensional alterations of the ridge following flapless tooth extraction in the anterior maxilla. Clinical Oral Implants Research. 2017;**28**(8):931-937

[46] Morton D, Chen ST, Martin WC, Levine RA, Buser D. Consensus statements and recommended clinical procedures regarding optimizing esthetic outcomes in implant dentistry. The International Journal of Oral & Maxillofacial Implants. 2014;**29**(Suppl):216-220

[47] Chen ST, Darby IB, Reynolds EC. A prospective clinical study of non-submerged immediate implants: Clinical outcomes and esthetic results. Clinical Oral Implants Research. 2007; **18**:552-562

[48] Wang HL, Kiyonobu K, Neiva RF. Socket augmentation: Rationale and technique. Implant Dentistry. 2004;**13**:286-296

[49] Nemcovsky CE, Artzi Z, Moses O, Gelernter I. Healing of marginal defects at implants placed in fresh extraction sockets or after 4–6 weeks of healing. A comparative study. Clinical Oral Implants Research. 2002;**13**:410-419

[50] Tarnow DP, Magner AW, Fletcher P. The effect of the distance from the contact point to the crest of bone on the presence or absence of the interproximal dental papilla. Journal of Periodontology. 1992;**63**:995-996

[51] Yalcin S, Aktas I, Emes Y, Kaya G, Aybar B, Atalay B. A technique for atraumatic extraction of teeth before immediate implant placement using implant drills. Implant Dentistry. 2009;**18**(6):464-472

[52] Rosenquist B, Grenthe B. Immediate placement of implants into extraction sockets: Implant survival. The International Journal of Oral & Maxillofacial Implants. 1996;**112**: 205-209

[53] Wilson TG Jr, Schenk R, Buser D, Cochran D. Implants placed in immediate extraction sites: A report of histologic and histometric analyses of human biopsies. The International Journal of Oral & Maxillofacial Implants. 1998;**133**:333-341

[54] Schropp L, Kostopoulos L, Wenzel A. Bone healing following immediate versus delayed placement of titanium implants into extraction sockets: A prospective clinical study. The International Journal of Oral & Maxillofacial Implants. 2003;**182**:189-199

[55] Yukna RA. Clinical comparison of hydroxyapatite-coated titanium dental implants placed in fresh extraction sockets and healed sites. Journal of Periodontology. 1991;**62**:468-472

[56] Gelb DA. Immediate implant surgery: Three year retrospective evaluation of 50 consecutive cases. The International Journal of Periodontics & Restorative Dentistry. 1993;**8**:388-399

[57] Becker W, Becker BE, Polizzi G, Bergström C. Autogenous bone grafting of bone defects adjacent to implants placed into immediate extraction sockets in patients: A prospective study. The International Journal of Oral & Maxillofacial Implants. 1994;**94**:389-396

[58] Lang NP, Bragger U, Hammerle CHF. Immediate transmucosal I mplants using the principle of guided tissue regeneration (GTR). I. Rationale, clinical procedures and 2 ½-year results. Clinical Oral Implants Research. 1994;**5**:154-163

[59] Edel A. The use of a connective tissue graft for closure over an immediate implant with an occlusive membrane. Clinical Oral Implants Research. 1995;**6**:60-65

[60] Wagenberg BD, Froum SJ. Implant complications related to immediate implant placement into extraction sites. In: Froum SJ, editor. Dental Implant Complications: Etiology, Prevention, and Treatment, 2nd ed. Hoboken, New Jersey: John Wiley & Sons; 2016. p. 457-479

[61] Araujo MG, Sukekava F, Wennstrom JL, Lindhe J. Ridge alterations following implant placement in fresh extraction sockets: An experimental study in the dog. Journal of Clinical Periodontology. 2005;**32**:645-652

[62] Araujo MG, Lindhe J. Dimensional ridge alterations following tooth extraction. An experimental study in the dog. Journal of Clinical Periodontology. 2005;**32**:212-218

[63] Quirynen M, Assche NV, Botticelli D, Berglundh T. How does timing of implant placement to extraction affect outcome? The International Journal of Oral & Maxillofacial Implants. 2007;**22**(Suppl):203-223

[64] Levine SS, Prewett AB, Cook SD. The use of a new form of allograft bone in implantation or osseointegrated dental implants—A preliminary report. The Journal of Oral Implantology. 1992;**18**:366-371

[65] Nordin T, Nilsson R, Frykholm A, Hallman M. A 3-arm study of early loading of rough-surfaced implants in the completely edentulous maxilla and in the edentulous posterior

maxilla and mandible: Results after 1 year of loading. The International Journal of Oral & Maxillofacial Implants. 2004;**19**:880-886

[66] Hammerle CH, Lang NP. Single stage surgery combining transmucosal implant placement with guided bone regeneration and bioresorbable materials. Clinical Oral Implants Research. 2001;**12**:9-18

[67] Langstaff WN. Immediate replacement of nonrestorable roots. The Journal of Oral Implantology. 2001;**27**:311-316

[68] Locante WM. The nonfunctional immediate provisional in immediate extraction sites: A technique to maximize esthetics. Implant Dentistry. 2001;**10**:254-258

[69] Sevor JJ, Meffert R. Placement of implants into fresh extraction sites using a resorbable collagen membrane: Case reports. Practical Periodontics and Aesthetic Dentistry. 1992;**4**: 35-41

[70] Pecora G, Andreana S, Covani U, De Leonardis D, Schifferle RE. New directions in surgical endodontics: Immediate implantation into an extraction socket. Journal of Endodontia. 1996;**223**:135-139

[71] Novaes AB Jr, Marcaccini AM, Souza SL, Taba M Jr, Grisi MF. Immediate placement of implants into periodontally infected sites in dogs: A histomorphometric study of bone implant contact. The International Journal of Oral & Maxillofacial Implants. 2003;**183**:391-398

Clinical Application of DDM/rhBMP-2 in Implant Dentistry

In-Woong Um, Young-Kyun Kim, Pil-Young Yun,
Zi-Yu Yan and Yu-Mi Kim

Additional information is available at the end of the chapter

http://dx.doi.org/10.5772/intechopen.79871

Abstract

Recombinant human bone morphogenetic protein-2 (rhBMP-2) is well-known osteoinductive growth factors that can be used along with various carriers. Demineralized dentin matrix (DDM) that has osteoinductive and osteoconductive capacities was developed as potential candidate for rhBMP-2 carrier that has its endogenous growth factors and fulfils the requirements such as controlled release kinetics, biocompatibility, biodegradabilities and bone forming capacity. DDM loaded with rhBMP-2 (DDM/rhBMP-2) have been subjected to in vitro, in vivo studies for the purpose of proving the clinical safety and efficacy. Recently the clinical trials and outcomes of DDM/rhBMP-2 have also proved this composite to be safe and efficient in terms of enhanced bone formation, remodeling capacity and reduced concentration of rhBMP-2 in implant dentistry in Korea. This chapter will introduce the clinical application of DDM/rhBMP-2 in implant dentistry based on the related experimental and clinical researches.

Keywords: demineralized dentin matrix (DDM), recombinant human bone morphogenetic protein-2 (rhBMP-2), DDM loaded with rhBMP-2 (DDM/rhBMP-2), bone graft, bone regeneration

1. Introduction

Since the first report of clinical application of DDM (AutoBT® Korea Tooth Bank, Seoul, Korea) that were developed by Korea Tooth Bank in 2010, many experimental and clinical studies have been subjected to improve the biocompatibility, bone forming capacity and to expand clinical applications.

DDM is fabricated from the tooth that is traditionally discarded after extraction as medical waste product. Based on the historical work of Dr. Urist since 1965 [1], DDM itself can be defined as acid insoluble, microporous, type I collagenous scaffold that has several non-collagenous growth factors such as BMPs, PDGF and FGF2 in addition to a mineral phase [2–4]. DDM is mainly processed by dehydration, defatting, and partial demineralization. Demineralization with 0.6 N HCl results in the elimination of the major part of the mineral phase and immunogenic components, while retaining a very low fraction of minerals (5–10 wt.%), the majority of Type I collagen, and non-collagenous proteins (NCPs), providing an osteoconductive and osteoinductive scaffold [5, 6].

We developed two types of DDM (AutoBT®): one is powder, the other is block. The clinical efficacy and safety of DDM powder and block have been approved as new health technology assessment (nHTA) in Korea 2015 based on the several experimental and clinical evidences [7–11].

DDM powder, which is proved to be osteoinductive and osteoconductive, is 300–800μm size with enlarged dentinal tubules and loosened collagen matrix that serve as channels for releasing essential growth factors from the dentin matrix. The indications of powder are socket preservation, alveolar bone augmentation, guided bone regeneration and sinus augmentation [12].

DDM block, which is osteoconductive and osteoinductive, is root form shaped and has several 200–300 μm-sized macropores from surface to pulp chamber and canal to provide a space for vascular invasion from the host tissues when implanted in the alveolar bone. The indication of block are socket preservation, alveolar wall repair and replacement of conventional membranes [11].

The rhBMP-2 was well known cytokines that has great potential of stimulation, proliferation, and differentiation of stem cells into osteoblastic cells to deposit newly formed osteoid. It has been shown that rhBMP-2 requires suitable carrier to achieve clinical efficacy. Suitable carriers should meet some requirements such as adequate porosity to allow cell and blood vessel infiltration, appropriate mechanical stability against compression and tension, biocompatibility, biodegradability, amenability to sterilization, adhesiveness to adjacent bone, affinity for BMPs, and should provide retention of the protein for a sufficient period of time to affect the repair [13].

Type I collagen (absorbable collagen sponge, ACS) is the most preferred and commonly used BMP carrier. In 2007, the FDA granted approval of rhBMP-2/ACS (INFUSE Bone Graft®, Medtronics, Memphis, TN) as an alternative to autogenous bone grafts for sinus augmentations, and for localized alveolar ridge augmentation of defects associated with extraction sockets. Dose dependent clinical studies have determined 1.5mg/cc as a safe and predictable dose for bone formation. However, the only approved carrier for rhBMP-2 by the US FDA at this time has many drawbacks such as poor mechanical properties, squeezing tendency of rhBMP-2 resulting in burst release and overdose complication, and less osteoconductivities. So that ideal rhBMP-2 carrier has not been established yet in field of clinical implant dentistry [14–16].

DDM has been considered as one of the potential candidate of the rhBMP-2 carrier in perspectives of the main role that is to retain the factor at the site for a prolonged period of time [17]. Regarding to DDM as rhBMP-2 carrier, Ike et al. reported that exogenous rhBMP-2 adsorbed into pulverized root partially demineralized dentin matrix (PDM) proved to be as osteoinductive as autogenous bone graft [18]. Murata et al. also showed that human DDM particles are osteoinductive, insoluble collagenous matrices, and DDMs might be effective as an rhBMP-2 carrier for bone engineering [19].

Based on the previous report of Ike and Murata, Kim et al. [20] and Um et al. [21] have reported and confirmed *in vivo* and *in vitro* studies that support the observations of efficacy of DDM as rhBMP-2 carrier. With regard to clinical applications, Kim reported the first successful use of DDM/rhBMP-2 in humans in 2014, while allogenic DDM/rhBMP-2 was successfully applied for upper right alveolar bone repair in 2016 [22].

Jeon et al. reported the evaluation of soft tissue volume change after socket preservation using DDM/rhBMP-2 compared with Bio-Oss collagen (Geistlich, Wolhusen, Switzerland) that the volume decreases of DDM/rhBMP-2 is not inferior to Bio-Oss [23].

Another clinical study of a total of 23 patients who received DDM/rhBMP-2 with implant placements (36 implants; maxilla: 14, mandible: 22) showed favorable osseointegration in terms of the implant stability, marginal bone loss, and clinical outcomes [24].

Recently, the author reported a clinical study of DDM/rhBMP-2 application on extraction socket preservation that DDM may be potential carrier of rhBMP-2 with reduced concentration of rhBMP-2 [25]. This chapter will introduce the surgical technique, clinical outcome, long term results of DDM/rhBMP-2 graft in implant dentistry.

2. Case reports

2.1. Preparation of DDM/rhBMP-2

DDM powder was produced using human teeth that were soaked in 70% ethyl alcohol. After dividing the teeth into the crown and root, the root portion was crushed to a powder. The size of the particles was between 300 and 800 μm diameter. The crushed particles were soaked in distilled water and a hydrogen dioxide solution, and the remaining foreign substances were removed by using an ultrasonic cleaner. The cleaned particles were dehydrated with ethyl alcohol and went through defatting using ethyl ether solutions. The particles were then demineralized for 30 min in 0.6 N HCl. The demineralized particles were lyophilized and sterilized with ethylene oxide gas (**Figure 1a**).

DDM block also was fabricated after crowns were severed at the cementoenamel junctions. Only root dentin part was processed for the block fabrication (European Patent No. 2462899) for its intended use as described in other report. [11] Additional holes sized in 0.2–0.3 mm were made from surface of the root to the canal area to create through and

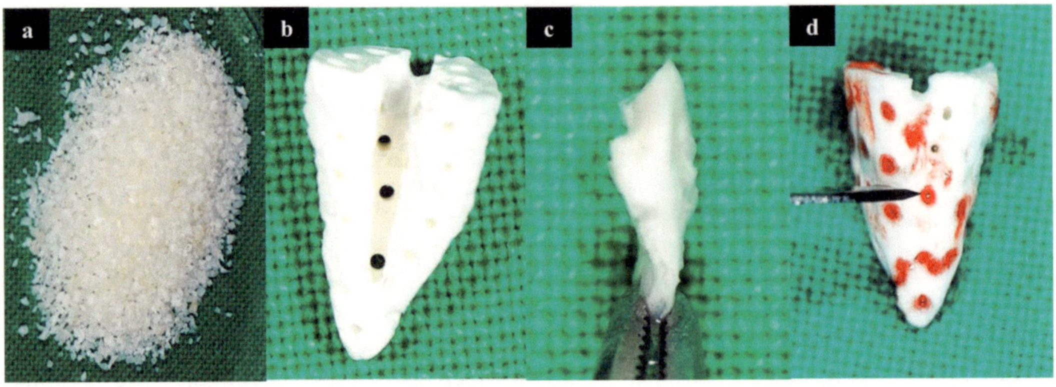

Figure 1. Types of DDM. (a) DDM powder; (b) DDM block with the through and through holes, 200–300μm diameter; (c) sheet like structure fabricated from block; (d) wettability with the blood via macropores.

through macropores for promoting vascular invasion and bone formation. The block went through the same fabrication process with the powder form, but the only difference was not being crushed into particles so that the block maintains the original tooth root form and shape (**Figure 1b**).

DDM block can be transformed into various shapes according to its indication such as sheet like structure to be membrane substitute, ring structure for vertical augmentation (**Figure 1c**). **Figure 1d** shows the characteristic wettability with patient's own blood via macropores of DDM block (**Figure 1d**).

The rhBMP-2 was loaded on the DDM powder and block by placing 5.0 μg of 0.2 mg/mL rhBMP-2 (Cowellmedi, Busan, Korea) and 0.3 g of DDM powder into individual 15-mL conical tubes. The mixtures were frozen in a deep freeze at −70°C for 60 min, slotted into a lyophilization glass bottle, and then fixed in a lyophilizer (ILShin Lab, Seoul, Korea). After sterilization with ethylene oxide, the DDM powder loaded with rhBMP-2 was packed and transported to the hospital where the implant surgery would be performed [22].

Because DDM/rhBMP-2 powder and block were manufactured in laboratory with maintaining its form and shape clinician can use this material simple and easy as usual.

Demographic information of patients, sites, procedure, materials and follow-up periods are summarized in **Table 1**.

Case No.	Age/Gender	Site	Procedure	Materials	Follow up
1	44 / F	Lower left first molar	SP /Simultaneous	Powder / No membrane	4 month
2	56 / F	Upper right first molar	SP / Simultaneous	Powder / No membrane	3 year 7 month
3	55 / F	Upper right central incisor	GBR /Simultaneous	Powder / No membrane	3 year
4	66 / F	Lower central incisors	Ridge split / Simultaneous	Powder / No membrane	3 year
5	54 / M	Lower left canine	GBR (alveolar) / Simultaneous	Powder / No membrane	3 year
6	43 / M	Lower left first molar	GBR / Staged	Block+Powder / No membrane	7 month
7	41 / M	Upper right first molar	Onlay / Simultaneous	Block+Powder / No membrane	7 year

F: Female, M: Male, SP: Socket prevention, GBR: Guided Bone Regeneration

Table 1. Demography of DDM/rhBMP-2 application.

2.2. DDM/rhBMP-2 powder

2.2.1. Case 1: socket preservation on lower left first molar extraction site with simultaneous implant placement

Implants were placed on the extraction socket of the lower left first molar (**Figure 2**) together with DDM/rhBMP-2 powder to prevent buccal wall resorption otherwise buccal wall collapse could hinder the dental implant management (**Figure 2a**). During the secondary surgery, 4 months post-implantation, sound bone and well organized tissues around the dental implant can be seen. DDM/rhBMP-2 powder seemed to be well incorporated with the extraction socket wall because both the border between the defect and DDM/rhBMP-2 particles was no longer visible (**Figure 2b**).

2.2.2. Case 2: socket preservation on upper right first molar with simultaneous implant placement

Implants was placed on the extraction socket of the upper right first molar (**Figure 3**) together with DDM/rhBMP-2 powder to prevent anticipated buccal wall resorption (**Figure 3a**). A cone beam computerized tomography (CBCT, Vatech, Seoul, Korea) image of the upper right first molar, taken three months after first surgery showed the graft which patched up the thin buccal cortical bone (**Figure 3b**). Six months post-implantation, i.e., at the time of secondary surgery, the buccal cortical bone seems to be resorbed and replaced with newly formed bone with the volume of socket wall maintained (**Figure 3c**). Three year seven months later with final prosthesis, the alveolar housing, surrounded dental implant, maintain its volume and shape as natural alveolar bone (**Figure 3d**).

Comparing 3D reconstructive images of immediate post operation to 3 year 7 months later indicated that the thin buccal cortical bone which was expected to be resorbed due to slightly

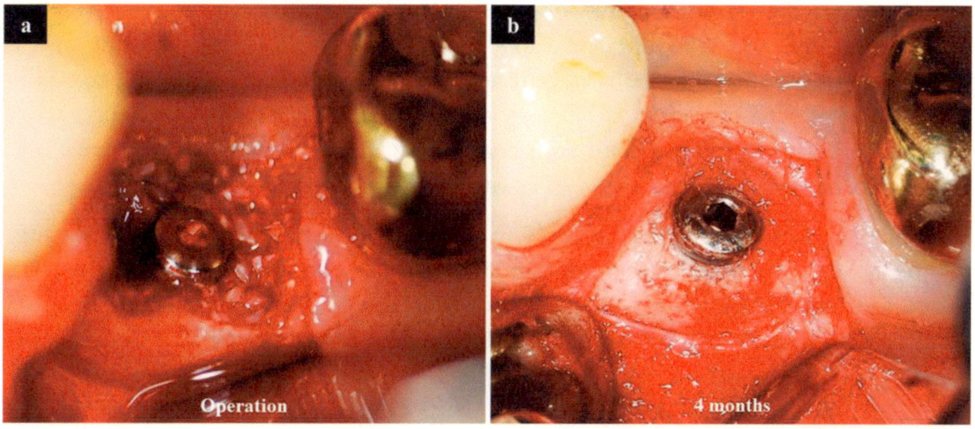

Figure 2. Socket preservation on lower left first molar without covering membrane. (a). Dental implant was placed in the extraction socket with primary stability, and the gap between the implant and socket wall was filled with DDM/rhBMP-2 powder without membrane. (b) Four months later, well organized bone was seen that surround the dental implant and repair all the gaps. Remnants of DDM/rhBMP-2 particles can not be seen.

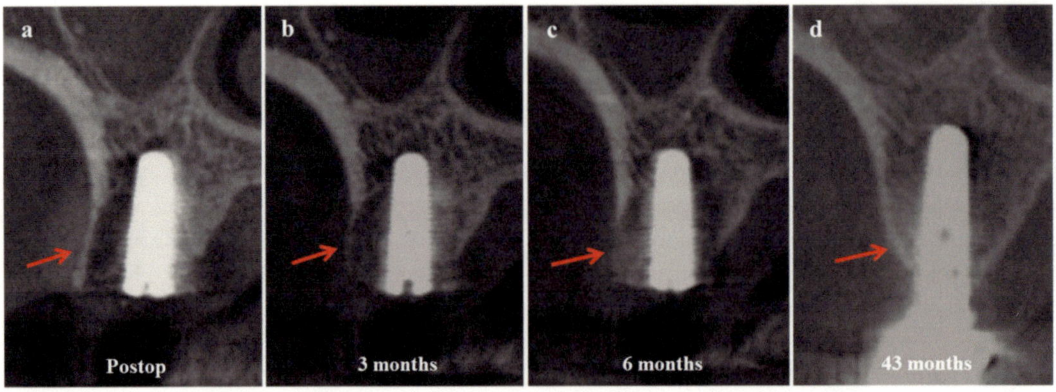

Figure 3. CBCT of socket preservation on upper right first molar with simultaneous implant placement. (a) Immediate postoperative image showed gap between the implant and thin buccal cortical bone which is expected to be resorbed. (b) Three months after graft, thinning buccal cortical bone indicated the beginning of remodeling. (c) Six months after graft, buccal cortical bone was almost disappeared with the volume of extraction socket maintained. (d) Three year 7 months after, alveolar bone around the dental implant turned into a mature cortical-cancellous bone complex (arrow = alveolar bone).

demineralized appearance (**Figure 4a**), and the alveolar bone surround the dental implant neck have been completely remodeled into a mature cortical bone which was fully supported by cancellous bone and marrow (**Figure 4b**).

2.2.3. Case 3: GBR on upper right central incisor

Upper right central incisor was extracted due to intermittent pain, swelling, and mobility for the past three years. One week after extraction, the implant (diameter: 3.8 mm, length: 13 mm; Dio, Busan, Korea) was placed and the DDM/rhBMP-2 was grafted simultaneously with securing excellent primary stability (**Figure 5a**).

The labial defect and exposed implant were covered with DDM/rhBMP-2 powders (**Figure 5b**). The muco-periosteal flap was replaced and stabilized without a covering membrane. After one and half months, the patient underwent secondary surgery earlier than the conventional waiting period of 6 months due to her inevitable schedule. Newly formed bone was covered the labial defect and exposed implant completely. The volume was maintained and the remained particles were no longer seen (**Figure 5c**).

A CBCT image taken before and immediately after the primary surgery showed the missing part of the labial cortex and exposed implant that had been patched up by the DDM/rhBMP-2 powder (**Figure 6a** and **b**). There were clear border lines separating the graft from the remaining labial cortex (**Figure 6b**). After 3 years with final prosthesis, the labial defect appeared completely repaired by sound cortico-cancellous bone. The border at the upper labial defect had completely disappeared, indicating good incorporation of the graft into the alveolar bone as well as remodeling capacity into sound cortico-cancellous bone complex around implant neck (**Figure 6c**).

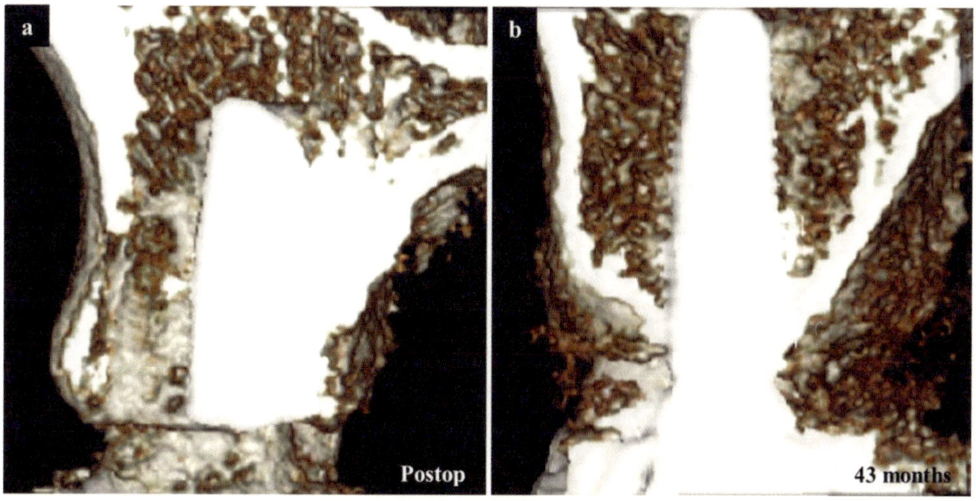

Figure 4. 3D reconstructive image from CBCT. (a) The demineralized buccal cortical bone which was expected to be resorbed. (b) The alveolar bone surround the implant neck have been completely remodeled into a mature cortico-cancellous bone complex.

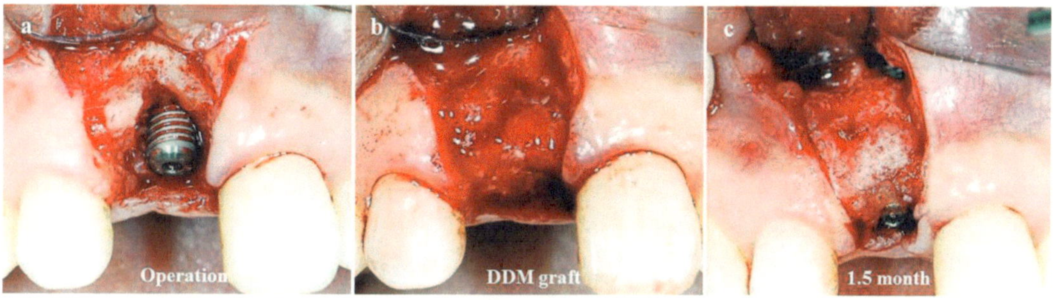

Figure 5. GBR on upper right central incisor. (a) Exposed dental implant and labial defect immediate after implant placement. (b) Exposed defect were covered with DDM/rhBMP-2 powders. See the wettability of DDM with blood that provides immobility to the powders without membrane. (c) Six weeks after, well organized, newly formed bones filled the labial defect and surround the dental implant.

2.2.4. Case 4: ridge split and expansion on lower central incisors

Ridge split procedure was performed to secure the labio-lingual dimension for implant placement (diameter: 3.8 mm, length: 13 mm; Daemul, Seoul, Korea) on lower central incisors (**Figure 7a**). The gaps created by ridge split and implant placement were filled with DDM/rhBMP-2 powders (**Figure 7b**). Two and a half months later, the whole DDM/rhBMp-2 particles have changed into well-organized bone-like structure with remarkably increased ridge width and height (**Figure 7c**). Well organized tissues covered screw was retrieved for histological examination (**Figure 7d**). There were no inflammatory cells or foreign body reactions and were no gaps between the DDM particle and the newly formed bone (**Figure 7e**).

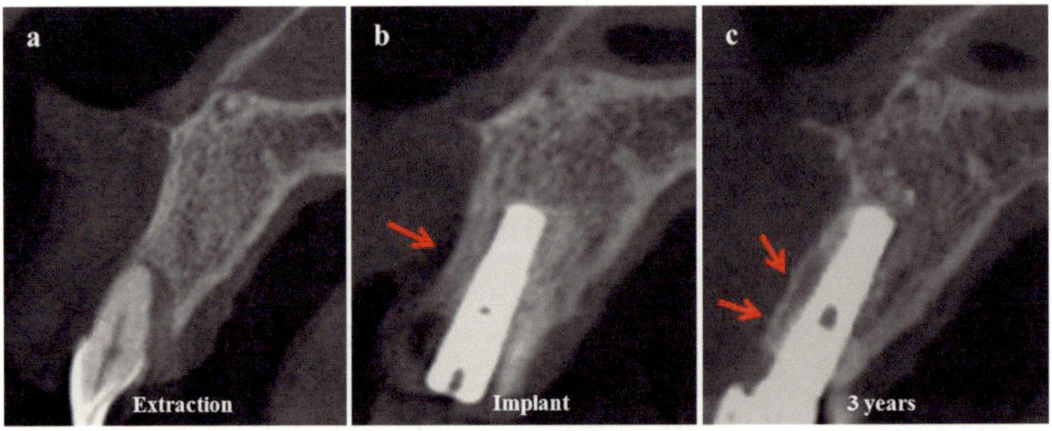

Figure 6. CBCT images of GBR on upper right central incisor. (a) Before extraction of upper right central incisor; (b) placement of dental implant and GBR was done for labial defect; (c) Three years follow up. The cortico-cancellous bone complex was recovered completely (arrow = alveolar bone).

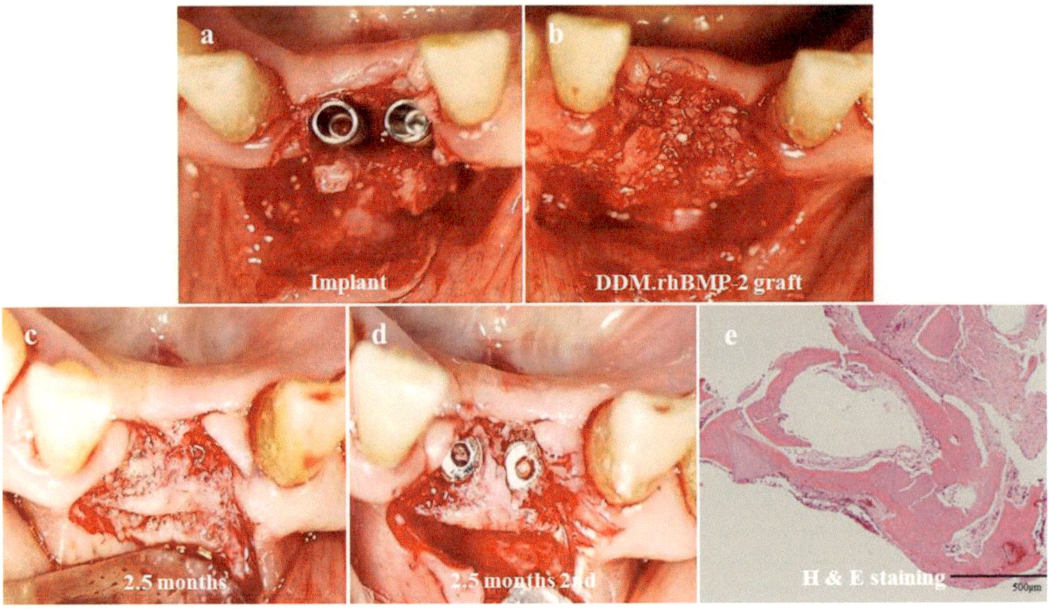

Figure 7. DDM/rhBMP-2 powder application on lower central incisors. (a) Implant placement after ridge split procedure. (b) The space between the implants and labial cortical plate is filled with DDM/rhBMP-2. No membrane is used. (c) Two and a half months later, a well-organized bone-like structure surrounded implant. The ridge width increased remarkably. (d) Uncovering implant. Tissue over the implant is used for histological evaluation. (e) Histologic specimen shows active new bone formation around DDM particle. Void space is the DDM which was detached during histologic processing. (Hematoxylin and eosin staining, Scale bar = 5.0 μm). From Um et al. [22] (**Figure 3**).

Histologic specimens of DDM alone at this area have shown that the particle was surrounded by a dense fibrotic capsule consisting of 3–4 cell layers where there are no inflammatory cells or foreign body reactions as the evidences of biocompatibility of DDM due to the environmental factors of poor blood supply in between the cover screw and the gingiva, we could not find the bone formation at this area before. [22] However, DDM/rhBMP-2 specimen in this case showed remarkable amount of bone formation around DDM/rhBMP-2 particles (**Figure 7e**). This may be explained by the positive effect of additional rhBMP-2 on DDM.

A CBCT image taken seven months after surgery showed a completely repaired labial bone. The demarcated border between the remaining labial cortex and the repaired bone has almost disappeared (**Figure 8a** and **b**). After 3 years with final prosthesis, the labial cortex becomes more thickened and fully supported by cancellous bone and marrow (**Figure 8c**).

2.2.5. Case 5: alveolar bone augmentation on lower left canine

Extraction of canine, which were sent to Korea Tooth Bank for fabrication of DDM/rhBMP-2, were performed one week before implant placement. Full thickness flaps were elevated to expose the alveolar crest and locate the defective area. Cleaning and removal of the granulation tissues revealed a huge, crater-like defect with complete destruction of the labial wall (**Figure 9a**). The implant (diameter: 3.8 mm, length: 13 mm; Dio, Busan, Korea) was placed and an excellent primary stability was obtained (**Figure 9b**). The huge defect and exposed implant were filled and augmented with DDM/rhBMP-2 that was prepared for easy molding and shaping (**Figure 9c**). The DDM/rhBMP-2 was placed and carefully packed into the destroyed area of the lingual wall and extended to the surface of the lateral buccal wall, without applying excessive pressure. The mucoperiosteal flap was replaced without a covering membrane (**Figure 9d**).

When the patient underwent secondary surgery, six months later, well-formed bone, which surrounds the implant and fill the gap, can be seen (**Figure 9e**). All routine prosthetic procedures after removal of bone over cover screw were performed (**Figure 9f**).

A CBCT image taken immediately after surgery showed that the missing part of the labial cortex had been patched up by the DDM/rhBMP-2 powder. There was clear border line

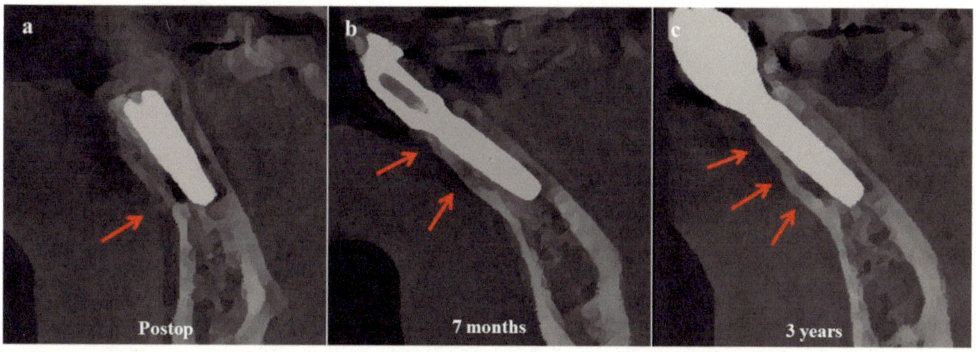

Figure 8. Cone beam computerized tomography (CBCT) of DDM/rhBMP-2 application on lower central incisor. (a) Immediately after implant placement and DDM/rhBMP-2 graft. There is obvious lower labial defect. (b) After 7 months. Labial cortical bone is completely repaired and the demarcated defect border has almost disappeared. (c) After 3 years. The labial cortex becomes thicker and shows fully developed cortico-cancellous bone complex (arrow = alveolar bone). From Um et al. [22] (**Figure 4**).

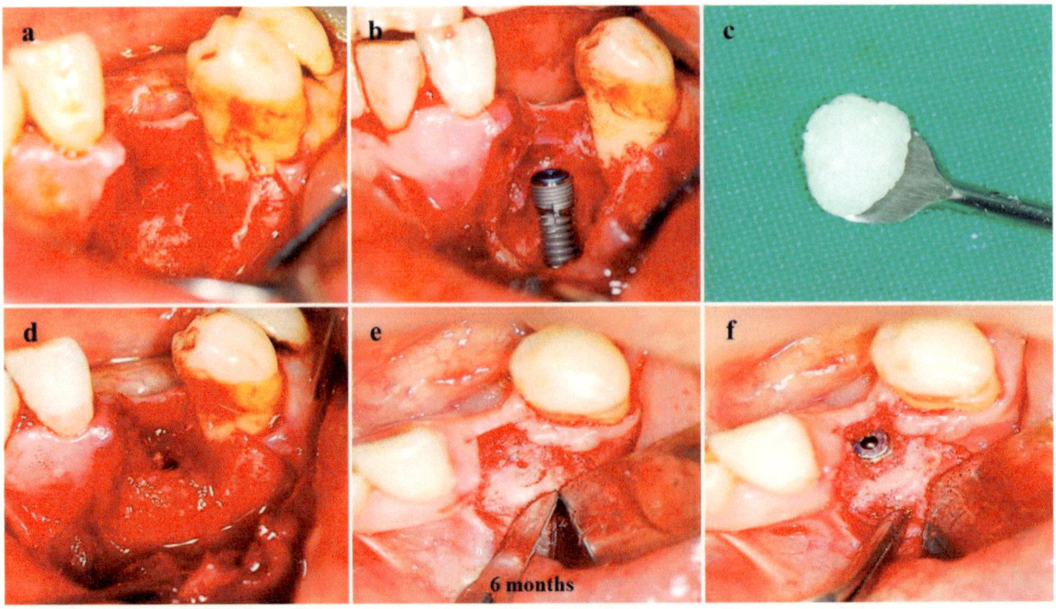

Figure 9. DDM/rhBMP-2 application on lower left canine. (a). There was huge defect after removal of all granulations on lower left canine. (b). Placement of implant (diameter: 3.8 mm, length: 13 mm) ensuring initial stability. (c). DDM/rhBMP-2 particles can be molded and shaped easily. (d). DDM/rhBMP-2 is packed into the lingual wall gap and along the labial wall. No membrane is used. (e). Well-organized bone tissue was found, filling the gap and surround the implant completely. None of the particles can be seen. (f). The tissue over the cover screw is typically removed in order to go through the prosthetic procedure and histological evaluation. From Um et al. [22] (**Figure 1**).

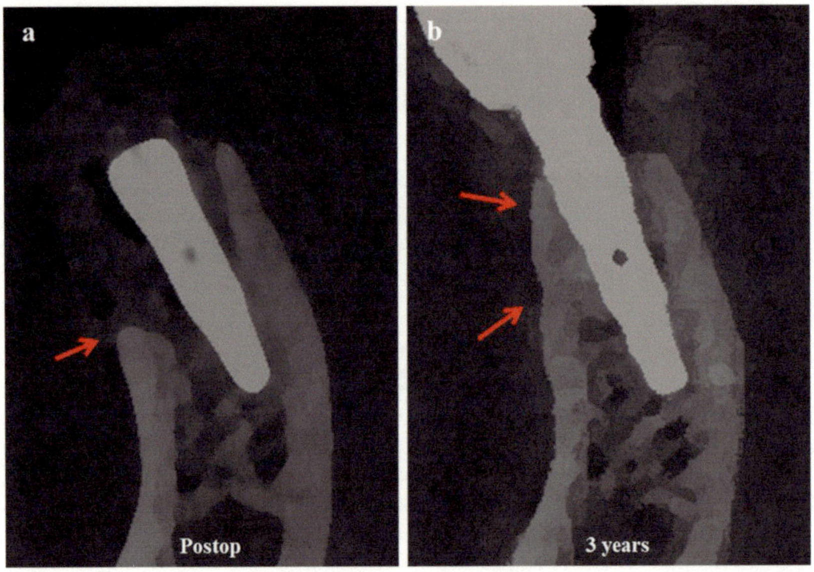

Figure 10. Cone beam computerized tomography (CBCT) of lower left canine repaired by DDM/rhBMP-2. (a) Immediately after implant placement and graft. DDM/rhBMP-2 particles surround the implant, patching up the labial and crestal alveolar bone. (b) After 3 years, the border line at the lower labial defect has completely disappeared. The repaired labial cortical bone was fully supported by cancellous bone and marrow (arrow = alveolar bone). From Um et al. [22] (**Figure 2**).

separating the graft from the remaining labial cortex (**Figure 10a**). After three years with final prosthesis, the alveolar bone was repaired completely in both volume and shape. The border at the lower labial defect had completely disappeared, indicating good incorporation of the graft into the alveolar bone. The repaired labial cortical bone seemed to be fully supported by cancellous bone and marrow (**Figure 10b**).

2.3. DDM/rhBMP-2 block

2.3.1. Case 1: GBR for the repair of alveolar wall on lower left first molar

After extraction of lower left first molar, there was collapsed buccal wall resulting in huge, crater-like defect (**Figure 11a** and **b**). Using the extracted tooth, block and powder type DDM/rhBMP-2 were prepared (**Figure 11c**). Buccal wall was repaired by block and the alveolar proper was repaired by powder (**Figure 11d**). Six months later for the staged procedure of implant placement, there was a bone-like tissue that was completely transformed from the block and powder of DDM/rhBMP-2. Alveolar bone seemed to be repaired completely without any remnants of block and powder (**Figure 11e**). So that the implant can be secured safely on the repaired alveolar bone (**Figure 11f**).

A CBCT image taken before and after extraction showed complete loss of buccal wall (**Figure 12a** and **b**). The alveolar proper was repaired by DDM/rhBMP-2 powder while the missing part of buccal wall was repaired by DDM/rhBMP-2 block. There was clear border line separating the block graft from the remaining buccal cortical bone (**Figure 12c**). After 6 months, the border line began to disappear that indicate good incorporation and remodeling

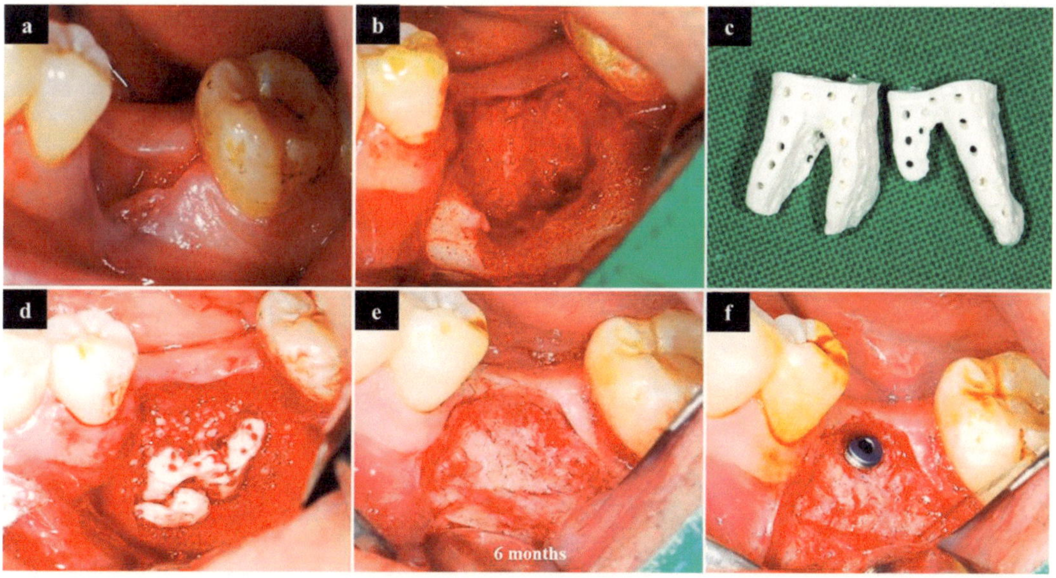

Figure 11. GBR for the repair of alveolar wall on lower left first molar. (a) Collapsed buccal wall after extraction of lower left first molar. (b) Reflection of flap and removal of granulation tissues. Huge defect and resorbed buccal wall can be seen. (c) Fabricated DDM/rhBMP-2 block from extracted tooth. (d) The huge defect was repaired by DDM/rhBMP-2 block and powder. (e) Six months later, whole DDM/rhBMP-2 was completely transformed into bone like structure. (f) Implant placement (staged procedure).

(**Figure 12d**), and 12 months later, radiopaque outer cortex and remodeled powder can be seen (**Figure 12e**). The alveolar bone surround the implant appeared completely repaired in both volume and shape.

2.3.2. Case 2: onlay graft on upper right first molar for volume expansion

After placement of implant, there was an atrophy of buccal cortical area (**Figure 13a**). DDM/rhBMP-2 block and powder was put on the buccal resorbed area that showed sound wettability with patients own blood and immobilization. The color change of the DDM/rhBMP-2 is mainly due to soaking with the patient's own blood into the macropores and collagenous dentin matrix (**Figure 13b**). Flap was closed without using membrane. The flap reflected again for the prosthetic procedure 4 months later, there were no discernible block and powders remained and well organized tissues replaced the onlay graft with the volume and shape maintained (**Figure 13c** and **d**).

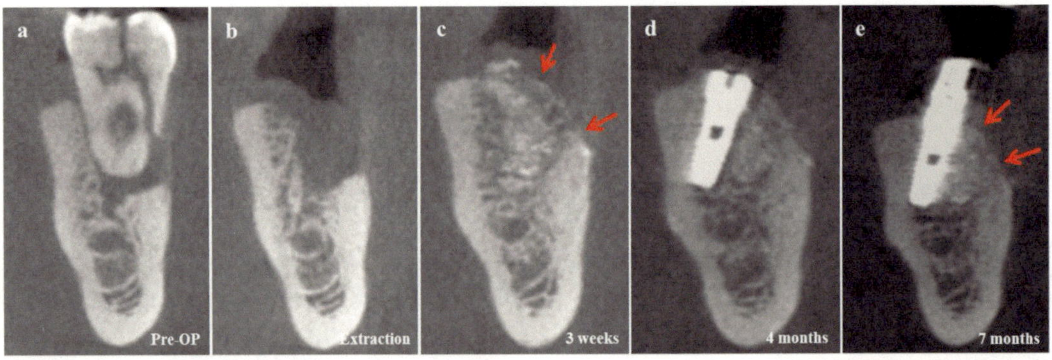

Figure 12. GBR for the repair of alveolar wall on lower left first molar. (a) Before extraction. (b) Immediate after extraction. Complete loss of buccal wall can be seen. (c) Repair the alveolar proper with DDM/rhBMP-2 powder and the buccal wall with DDM/rhBMP-2 block. (d) Six months later, placement of implant. See the remodeled powder. (e) Seven months after. Powders are remodeled in the alveolar proper, while the block repaired buccal cortical bone (arrow = alveolar bone).

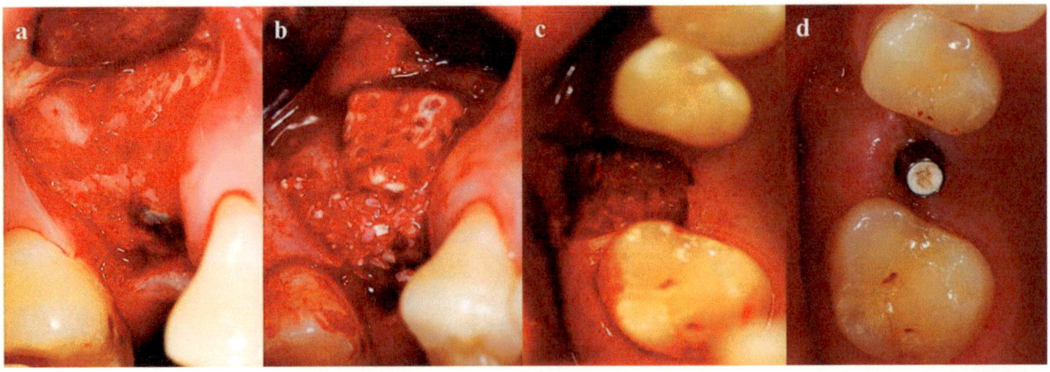

Figure 13. Onlay graft on upper right first molar for volume expansion. (a) Atrophied buccal area can be seen after placement of implant. (b) DDM/rhBMP-2 block and powder were put on the buccal resorbed area. No membrane was used due to the wettability of block and power with patient's own blood resulting in immobilization. (c) Four months later, there were no DDM particles and block that have changed into well-organized tissues maintaining the whole volume of DDM/rhBMP-2. (d) See the increased volume of buccal gingiva and texture.

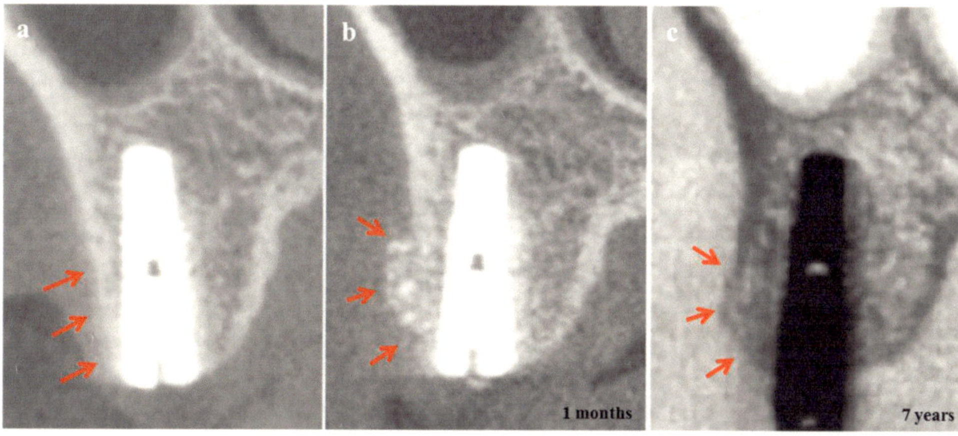

Figure 14. CBCT images of onlay graft on upper right first molar. (a) After placement of 3.8 mm diameter implant, the buccal cortical bone around the dental implant is too thin and close to implant neck. (b) Increased alveolar bone volume around implant neck area by DDM/rhBMP-2 application can be seen. (c) Seven years later, onlay DDM/rhBMP-2 was well incorporated with the buccal cortical bone under continuous remodeling, that create new cortico-cancellous bone complex (arrow = alveolar bone).

CBCT images after implant placement on upper right first molar. As a result of long term missing of tooth, alveolar ridge became narrow and the buccal cortical bone around the dental implant is too thin and close to implant neck (**Figure 14a**). Increased alveolar bone width and volume by DDM/rhBMP-2 application can be seen (**Figure 14b**). Seven years later, increased volume of alveolar housing, remodeled completely, shows mature cortico-cancellous bone complex (**Figure 14c**).

3. Discussion

Unlike other scaffolds, for example, ACS which has a limited capacity for controlled release, lacks of structural stability, risk of physiologically excessive doses, and the insufficient retention of BMP-2 [14–16], DDM has adequate porosity to allow cell and blood vessel infiltration, appropriate mechanical stability to withstand compression and tension, biocompatibility, biodegradability, amenability to sterilization, adhesiveness to adjacent bone, affinity for BMPs, and the ability to retain the protein for a sufficient period [17, 26]. DDM has a microporous structure with dentinal tubules 3–5 μm in diameter, which allows it not only to contain BMPs, but also to efficiently release them at surgical site [20]. Numerous studies have reported on the performance of DDM as a scaffold for BMPs; the osteoconductive and osteoinductive abilities of DDM are deemed to be its greatest strengths [18–20].

3.1. Experimental studies of DDM/rhMP-2

As a candidate for an rhBMP-2 carrier, Ike et al. reported that xenogenous rhBMP-2 adsorbed into pulverized root and partially DDM proved to be as osteoinductive as an autogenous bone graft [18]. Murata also showed that human DDM particles are osteoinductive, insoluble collagenous matrices, and that DDMs might be effective as an rhBMP-2 carrier for bone engineering [19].

The first report of human DDM/rhBMP-2 have demonstrated that DDM displays the highest released to loaded rhBMP-2 ratio, the lowest release speed, and the highest induction of osteonectin expression, resulting in augmented mature bone formation compare with tricalcium phosphate (TCP) [12]. Um et al. examined the bone induction capacity of DDM/ rhBMP-2 compare with conventional TCP in the muscle pouches of nude mice. The results were that the early cellular reaction on the surface of particles was superior in the DDM/ rhBMP-2 group, more osteoid was deposited on the DDM/ rhBMP-2 group [25].

In the rabbit's calvarial defect, the DDM and anorganic bovine bone combined with rhBMP-2 (ABB/rhBMP-2) groups showed osteoconductive bone formation, while the DDM/rhBMP-2 group showed osteoconductive and osteoinductive bone formation. The DDM/rhBMP-2 group showed a twofold greater amount of bone formation compared to the DDM alone and ABB/rhBMP-2 groups. The μCT analysis showed markedly increased bone volume in the DDM/rhBMP-2 group at eight weeks compared with that of the DDM group [21]. Kim et al. evaluated the efficacy of DDM/rhBMP-2 in the unilateral upper second and third premolars of eight beagles compare with the autogenous bone and reported equality of DDM/rhBMP-2 to autogenous bone [24].

3.2. Clinical studies of DDM/ rhBMP-2

Case series study of comparing short term outcome of DDM/rhBMP-2 (Bioα, Seongnam, Korea) with hydroxyapatite (HA)/rhBMP-2 (Bioα, Seongnam, Korea), reported that rhBMP-2 combined with HA or DDM scaffolds can be used for bone graft procedures such as guided bone regeneration [20].

About the effectiveness of DDM/rhBMP-2 (CowellMedi, Busan, Korea) for alveolar bone repair [27, 28], the clinical findings with respect to the healing process were that there were no remarkable inflammation and immune rejection that impair the healing process and are coincident with those of the previous studies of DDM alone [8, 10, 29]. The nanopore structure of dentinal tubules in unique avascular and acellular Type I collagenous dentin matrix seems to make it feasible to carry and release rhBMP-2 effectively on local site based on the previous study [30, 31].

In the clinical study of histological comparison of autogenous and allogenic DDM/rhBMP-2 at the site between the implant cover screw and gingiva, as the poor blood supply allows it to simulate a heterotopic condition, three patients undergoing simultaneous implant placement and receiving a different type of graft were included: allogenic DDM loaded with rhBMP-2 (DDM/rhBMP-2), autogenous DDM/rhBMP-2 and autogenous DDM. After 3–6 months of grafts, the antigenicity and immunogenicity of the carrier allogenic DDMs are low enough to maintain both the biocompatibility of the scaffold and the activity of the loaded rhBMP-2 [22].

Jeon et al. reported study to evaluate soft tissue volume change after socket preservation using DDM alone, DDM/rhBMP-2 and Bio-Oss collagen (Geistlich, Wolhusen, Switzerland). According to soft tissue volume changes, each groups showed statistically meaningful volume decreases. Bio-Oss collagen showed 15.4% volume decrease, DDM showed 18.8% and DDM/rhBMP-2 showed 16.1% decrease, respectively. However, there were no significant differences among groups [23].

In the clinical study of a total of 23 patients who received bone grafts using human DDM/rhBMP-2 with implant placements (36 implants; maxilla: 14, mandible: 22). The implant stability, marginal bone loss, and clinical outcome were evaluated. Favorable osseointegration was obtained in 35 out of 36 implant sites (one case of osseointegration failure) and severe complications were not observed in all cases [24].

3.3. Case report of DDM/ rhBMP-2

Each case report represent socket preservation, GBR, ridge split and expansion, onlay graft with simultaneous or staged implant placement. Besides the crucial factors for implant success such as stability, peri-implantitis, the first critical observation in this case presentation is the texture of tissues formed around the implant at second surgery time without using any membranes. The powder or block that were no longer visible when the flap reflected at 3–6 months after graft indicated good incorporation and remodeling capacities of DDM into host bed. These phenomena might be explained by the synergistic effect of exogenous rhBMP-2 with endogenous growth factors in DDM that is both increased bone formation and accelerated DDM degradation. This is assumption raised and explained in the previous report [18, 19, 31].

Second observation is the structure of bone around the implant neck area where the major peri-implantitis start and accumulated. What we need for ideal osseointegration is sound alveolar bone with appropriate volume and shape at this defense front area. The sound alveolar bone consist of cortical bone with enough thickness, and cancellous bone with mature bone marrow that is inevitable for continuous remodeling with standing for occlusal forces. At least one year after final prosthesis, we found sound cortical bone supported by fully developed cancellous bone in CBCT analysis. And the time to achieve sound bone around the neck area might be faster than that of DDM alone [8].

Third observation is histologic evidences we presented recently that shows more bone formation at each time point and accelerated resorption of DDM compare to other carriers such as HA and TCP [25].

Finally, the rationale for not using membrane is that carrier DDM is a collagenous scaffold with minerals to be able to absorb enough blood resulting in space maintenance and invasion of blood vessels from the host. In the clinical study of DDM/rhBMP-2 application in on extraction socket preservation, there were no cellular invasion from gum tissues to hinder bone formation clinically and radiologically [25].

4. Conclusion

The clinical application of DDM/ rhBMP-2 showed successful alveolar socket preservation, GBR, onlay graft in implant dentistry without any complications. Furthermore, this clinical success may open the way to new technology for alveolar bone repair, even though the cases presented here are small numbers and not representative to conclude the clinical superiority compare to others. For example, because the long term data of DDM/rhBMP-2 in sinus augmentation are not established yet, we need to collect more data from well controlled prospective studies.

Based on several other reports that have shown favorable results from using DDM/rhBMP-2 in implant dentistry, we are going to perform more number of clinical studies such as prospective, randomized, controlled clinical trials for the purpose of assuring the safety and efficacy of DDM as a promising carrier for rhBMP-2.

By the application of rhBMP-2 from experimental researches to clinical reality, the number of choice of alternative bone graft substitutes has been increased in implant dentistry. Although significant effort has been made to find a safer, cheaper, and more efficient scaffold for rhBMP-2 carrier, there have not been sufficient studies and efforts that focused on the application of rhBMP-2 in dental field.

By the discovery and successful applications of DDM as rhBMP-2 carrier in implant dentistry, we might have cheaper, safer and more efficient bone graft substitute. Reduced concentration of rhBMP-2 with similar or superior efficacy in inducing bone formation without the adverse effects made the DDM/rhBMP-2 revolutionary cost-effective and safe that eliminates most of the side effects associated with supraphysiologic overdose concentration.

Up to date, the long term results of DDM/rhBMp-2 are clearly promising in biologic activities and cost-benefits for the patients that would open the door to develop DDM as carrier of stem cells to be applied in implant dentistry.

Acknowledgements

This study was provided the data by the Seoul National University Bundang Hospital, Peking University, and the In-Dental Clinic.

Conflict of interest

The authors have declared that no conflict of interests exists.

Author details

In-Woong Um[1*], Young-Kyun Kim[2], Pil-Young Yun[2], Zi-Yu Yan[3] and Yu-Mi Kim[1]

*Address all correspondence to: h-bmp@hanmail.net

1 R&D Institute, Korea Tooth Bank, Seoul, Republic of Korea

2 Department of Oral and Maxillofacial Surgery, Section of Dentistry, Seoul National University Bundang Hospital, Seongnam, Republic of Korea

3 Department of Oral and Maxillofacial Surgery, Peking University School and Hospital of Stomatology, Beijing, China

References

[1] Urist MR. Bone: Formation by autoinduction. Science. 1965;**150**:893-899

[2] Murata M. Collagen biology for bone regenerative surgery. Journal of the Korean Association of Oral and Maxillofacial Surgeons. 2012;**38**:321-325. DOI: 10.5125/jkaoms.2012.38.6.321

[3] Yeomans JD, Urist MR. Bone induction by decalcified dentine implanted into oral, osseous and muscle tissues. Archives of Oral Biology. 1967;**12**:999-1008. DOI: 10.1016/0003-9969(67)90095-7

[4] Kim YK, Lee JK, Kim KW, Um IW, Murata M. Advances in biomaterials science and biomedical applications. In: Pignatello R, editor. Healing Mechanism and Clinical Application of Autogenous Tooth Bone Graft Material. Catania: InTech; 2013. pp. 405-437. DOI: 10.5772/53200

[5] Kim YK, Lee JH, Kim KW, Um IW, Murata M, Ito K. Analysis of organic components and osteoinductivity in autogenous tooth bone graft material. Journal of the Korean Association of Maxillofacial Plastic and Reconstructive Surgeons. 2013;**35**:353-359. DOI: 10.14402/jkamprs.2013.35.6.353

[6] Kim YK, Kim SG, Yun PY, Yeo IS, Jin SC, Oh JS, Kim HJ, Yu SK, Lee SY, Kim JS, Um IW, Jeong MA, Kim GW. Autogenous teeth used for bone grafting: A comparison with traditional grafting materials. Oral Surgery, Oral Medicine, Oral Pathology, Oral Radiology. 2014;**117**:e39-e45. DOI: 10.1016/j.oooo.2012.04.018. Epub 2012 Aug 30

[7] Kim YK, Um IW, Murata M. Tooth bank system for bone regeneration—Safety report. Journal of Hard Tissue Biology. 2014;**23**:371-376. DOI: 10.2485/jhtb.23.371

[8] Kim YK, Lee JH, Um IW, Cho WJ. Guided Bone regeneration using demineralized dentin matrix: Long-term follow-up. Journal of Oral and Maxillofacial Surgery. 2016;**74**(3):515.e1-515.e9. DOI: 10.1016/j.joms.2015.10.030. Epub 2015 Nov 10

[9] Lee HJ, Hong JS, Kim YK, Um IW, Lee JI. Osteogenic potential of demineralized dentin matrix as bone graft material. Journal of Hard Tissue Biology. 2017;**26**:223-230. DOI: 10.2485/jhtb.26.223

[10] Pang KM, Um IW, Kim YK, Woo JM, Kim SM, Lee JH. Autogenous demineralized dentin matrix from extracted tooth for the augmentation of alveolar bone defect: A prospective randomized clinical trial in comparison with anorganic bovine bone. Clinical Oral Implants Research. 2017;**28**:809-815. DOI: 10.1111/clr.12885. Epub 2016 Jun 8

[11] Kim YK, Pang KM, Yun PY, Leem DH, Um IW. Long-term follow-up of autogenous tooth bone graft blocks with dental implants. Clinical Case Reports. 2017;**5**:108-118. DOI: 10.1002/ccr3.754. eCollection 2017 Feb

[12] Kim YK, Kim SG, Bae JH, Um IW, Oh JS, Jeong KI. Guided bone regeneration using autogenous tooth bone graft in implant therapy: Case series. Implant Dentistry. 2014;**23**(2):138-143. DOI: 10.1097/ID.0000000000000046

[13] Burg KJ, Porter S, Kellam JF. Biomaterial developments for bone tissue engineering. Biomaterials. 2000;**21**:2347-2359. DOI: 10.1016/S0142-9612(00)00102-2

[14] Benglis D, Wang MY, Levi AD. A comprehensive review of the safety profile of bone morphogenetic protein in spine surgery. Neurosurgery. 2008;**62**:ONS423-ONS431. DOI: 10.1227/01.neu.0000326030.24220.d8

[15] Ripamonti U, Duarte R, Ferretti C. Re-evaluating the induction of bone formation in primates. Biomaterials. 2014;**35**:9407-9422. DOI: 10.1016/j.biomaterials.2014.07.053. Epub 2014 Aug 23

[16] Seeherman H, Li R, Bouxsein M, Kim H, Li XJ, Smith-Adaline EA, Aiolova M, Wozney JM. rhBMP-2/calcium phosphate matrix accelerates osteotomy-site healing in a nonhuman primate model at multiple treatment times and concentrations. The Journal of Bone and Joint Surgery. American Volume. 2006;**88**:144-160

[17] Li RH, Wozney JM. Delivering on the promise of bone morphogenetic proteins. Trends in Biotechnology. 2001;**19**:255-265

[18] Ike M, Urist MR. Recycled dentin root matrix for a carrier of recombinant human bone morphogenetic protein. The Journal of Oral Implantology. 1998;**24**:124-132

[19] Murata M. Bone Engineering using human demineralized dentin matrix and recombinant human BMP-2. Journal of Hard Tissue Biology. 2005;**14**:80-81. DOI: 10.2485/jhtb.14.80

[20] Kim YK, Um IW, An HJ, Kim KW, Hong KS, Murata M. Effects of demineralized dentin matrix used as an rhBMP-2 carrier for bone regeneration. Journal of Hard Tissue Biology. 2014;**23**:415-422

[21] Um IW, Hwang SH, Kim YK, Kim MY, Jun SH, Ryu JJ, Jang HS. Demineralized dentin matrix combined with recombinant human bone morphogenetic protein-2 in rabbit calvarial defects. Journal of the Korean Association of Oral and Maxillofacial Surgeons. 2016;**42**:90-98. DOI: 10.5125/jkaoms.2016.42.2.90. Epub 2016 Apr 27

[22] Um IW, Jun SH, Yun PY, Kim YK. Histological comparison of autogenous and allogenic demineralized dentin matrix loaded with recombinant human bone morphogenetic protein-2 for alveolar bone repair: A preliminary report. Journal of Hard Tissue Biology. 2017;**26**:417-424. DOI: 10.2485/jhtb.26.417

[23] Jeon TH, Kang MH, Um IW, Ryu JJ, Jun SH. Volumetric assessment of alveolar bone ridge after socket preservation using 3-dimensional surface model analysis. The Korea Research Society for Dental Material. 2017;**44**:377-386. DOI: 10.14815/kjdm.2017.44.4.377

[24] Kim SY, Kim YK, Park YH, Park JC, Ku JK, Um IW, Kim JY. Evaluation of the healing potential of demineralized dentin matrix fixed with recombinant human bone morphogenetic protein-2 in bone grafts. Materials (Basel). 2017;**7**:10. DOI: 10.3390/ma10091049

[25] Um IW. Demineralized dentin matrix as a carrier of recombinant human morphogenetic proteins. In: Proceeding of the 59th Congress of Korean Association of Oral and Maxillofacial Surgeons (JKAOMS); 26-28 April 2018; Korea. Korea: ISSN; 2018. pp. 72-73

[26] Kirker-Head CA. Potential applications and delivery strategies for bone morphogenetic proteins. Advanced Drug Delivery Reviews. 2000;**43**:65-92

[27] Um IW, Cho WJ, Kim YK. Experimental study on human demineralized dentin matrix as rhBMP-2 carrier *in vivo*. Journal of Dental Applications. 2015;**2**:269-273

[28] Kim YK, Jang HJ, Um IW. A case report of allogenic demineralized dentin matrix loaded with recombinant human bone morphogenetic proteins for alveolar bone repair. Journal of Dental and Oral Health. 2016;**2**:45

[29] Kim YK, Kim SG, Byeon JH, Lee HJ, Um IU, Lim SC, Kim SY. Development of a novel bone grafting material using autogenous teeth. Oral Surgery, Oral Medicine, Oral Pathology, Oral Radiology, and Endodontics. 2010;**109**:496-503. DOI: 10.1016/j.tripleo.2009.10.017. Epub 2010 Jan 8

[30] Murata M, Sato D, Hino J, Akazawa T, Tazaki J, Ito K, Arisue M. Acid-insoluble human dentin as carrier material for recombinant human BMP-2. Journal of Biomedical Materials Research. Part A. 2012;**100**:571-577. DOI: 10.1002/jbm.a.33236. Epub 2011 Dec 30

[31] Um IW, Kim YK, Jun SH, Kim MY, Cui NH. Demineralized dentin matrix as a carrier of recombinant human bone morphogenetic proteins: *In vivo* study. Journal of Hard Tissue Biology. 2018;**27**:219-226

Section 3

Post Implant Placement - Cosmetics and Complications

Chapter 4

Abutment Selection for Anterior Implant-Supported Restorations

Pinar Turkoglu, Adnan Kose and Deniz Sen

Additional information is available at the end of the chapter

http://dx.doi.org/10.5772/intechopen.80965

Abstract

With the introduction of dental implants to the market, varying restorative options have been successfully added for restoring the function and esthetics of both completely and partially edentulous patients. Accurate prosthodontic rehabilitation is the key factor for providing the long-term success and the survival of osseointegrated implants. Implant-supported restorations can be fabricated with different techniques. The prefabricated abutments provided by the implant companies are accepted as the gold standard because of their biocompatibility and advanced mechanical properties. However, especially for the anterior restorations, they are increasingly being replaced by custom abutments ideally prepared with CAD/CAM techniques; due to disadvantages of prefabricated abutments such as esthetic flaws, mechanical insufficiency resulting from implant placement, unacceptable emergence profile, and unhygienic regions formed under angled abutments. Currently, custom abutments are reported to have functional and esthetic advantages over prefabricated abutments. In this chapter, indications for proper abutment selection, contemporary production techniques, and different abutment materials will be stated, and the current research on the subject will be discussed.

Keywords: abutment, CAD/CAM, emergency profile, hybrid abutment, zirconia

1. Introduction

Implant-supported restorations have become a popular treatment choice for the rehabilitation of the partially edentulous patients with missing teeth particularly in the anterior region, where esthetics has an irreplaceable importance in treatment success [1]. Accurate prosthodontic rehabilitation is the key factor for providing the long-term success and the survival of osseointegrated implants [2]. Implant-supported restorations can be fabricated with several techniques and materials [1, 2]. This chapter evaluates the historical development of abutment types, their usage, and the studies evaluating the survival rates of abutments used in the anterior restorations.

Abutment-crown complex for single-tooth restorations was first introduced in 1986 [1]. This one-piece complex was primarily composed of acrylic resin crown veneered onto prefabricated machined titanium [1, 2]. Subsequently, for obtaining better esthetics, this complex was changed to a two-piece restoration consisting of a cemented metal-ceramic crown that was supported by a prefabricated titanium abutment [1]. Afterward, the University of California Los Angeles (UCLA) abutment was introduced in 1988, which made it possible to use custom cast metal component that can be screwed into the implant [3]. This abutment type gained popularity in time and still continues to be preferred for both screw- and cement-retained implant-supported restorations.

Until today, a large number of clinical studies have displayed perfect survival rates for metal abutments used in both anterior and posterior regions [4–7]. However, metal abutments have some limitations and disadvantages, predominantly related with the esthetic results. Clinical studies reported that metal abutments caused a blue-grayish color reflection from the peri-implant site gingiva, which threatens the treatment success especially for the patients with a high/gummy smile line [8–11]. To solve the esthetic problems related with metal abutments, Prestipino and Ingber introduced a densely sintered alumina ceramic abutment in 1993 [12–14]. The development of alumina ceramic abutments parallel with the improvements in the CAD/CAM technology was an important breakthrough in implant dentistry that was investigated with a wide range of clinical studies [15]. Then, in 2004, a densely sintered yttrium-stabilized zirconia was described by Glauser et al. as an alternative abutment material to alumina [16]. At first, zirconia abutments were produced manually with copy-milling technique using a customized resin pattern. Since then, fabricating zirconia abutments with CAD/CAM system led to significant improvements in implant dentistry enabling the replacement of a missing anterior tooth with an implant supporting a restoration with ideal esthetics and function. Zirconia abutments were developed offering a large number of biological advantages in comparison with titanium: less bacterial adhesion [17] and more biocompatibility due to lack of corrosion and galvanic coupling [18, 19].

Use of CAD/CAM technology in the dental market allowed the fabrication of custom abutments that can be manufactured from either titanium or ceramics [20]. Currently, preparation of individual custom abutments is also possible in accordance with the patients' anatomic needs and/or with the ideal emergence profile of the missing tooth [21].

2. Classification of implant abutments

Varying types of implant abutments have been reported in the literature for use with the anterior implant-supported restorations [22]. They can be classified according to the connection method to the restoration, fabrication material, fabrication method, type of abutment-implant connection, and color (**Table 1**).

Category	Options
Method of connection to restoration	- Screw-retained abutment-crown complex
	- Two-piece design with screw-retained crown over the abutment
	- Two-piece design with cemented crown over the abutment
Abutment connection to implant	- External connection
	- Internal connection
Material	- Titanium
	- Cast metal (noble, high noble, or base metal alloy)
	- Cast metal with porcelain fused at the base
	- Alumina
	- Complete zirconia
	- Zirconia with a titanium base (zirconia-titanium hybrid abutment)
Method of fabrication	- Prefabricated (unmodified or modified)
	- Customized cast abutment
	- Customized copy-milled abutment
	- Customized CAD-CAM abutment
Color	- Gold
	- Silver (metallic finish)
	- Pure white
	- Customized white
	- Customized pink/gingival shade at the cervical region

Table 1. Classification of implant abutment designs [22].

Differing properties of the abutments have varying advantages and disadvantages. Occlusal forces with different vectors are significantly lower in the anterior teeth than the posterior teeth because of Class III lever system of the human jaw [23, 24]. When compared with the incisors, biting forces are almost two times higher for the premolar teeth and three times higher for the molar teeth. Consequently, the clinical results between anterior and posterior abutments should be importantly different. Furthermore, esthetic parameters related to the selection of an anterior abutment may not be applied to the posterior regions. The readers should be aware that studies investigating the clinical outcomes of prosthetic components are classified as anterior and posterior regions due to significantly different complications and survival rates [22].

2.1. Implant-abutment connections

The implant-abutment connections can be classified as either external, which protrudes above the implant platform, or internal, which sets down in the access hole inside the implant body (**Figure 1**). The external hex design was the first to be used in the manufacturing of dental implants. It was originally 0.7 mm in height and was used to help screw the implant fixture into the prepared osteotomy. It was not used as an antirotational device because the rotation of the

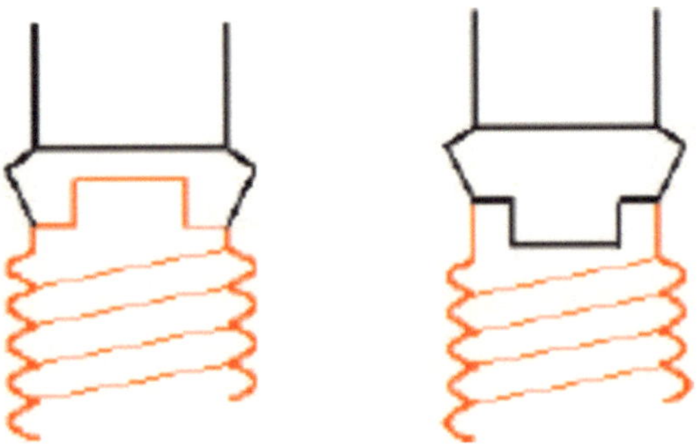

Figure 1. Schematic diagram of abutment-implant connection types [25].

implant-supported restoration was not an issue. However, when the dental implants began to be used in replacing a single-missing tooth, the external hex with some improved quality was used to prevent rotation of the abutment under loading. The external hex connection is still in use as it is suitable for the two-piece implant placement method, has an antirotational mechanism, and is compatible with different implant systems. The external hex also helps the laboratory technician to achieve the best possible emergence profile because the porcelain can be brought closer to the implant-abutment interface. However, it is not without disadvantages, such as low resistance for rotational and lateral movements owing to its high center of rotation. Furthermore, difficulty in seating the abutments in a deep gingival sulcus, increased screw loosening, and component fractures are problems to be considered when the external hex connectors are used [25].

The internal hex connector is widely used. It is a stable connection with a high resistance to lateral forces because of the lower center of rotation and is also suitable for a one-stage implant placement technique. It is also characterized by a good distribution of imposed force. However, weakening of the lateral wall of the implant at the connecting part and compensation for mismatching in the angle between implant fixtures may cause some problems [25].

There is a general consensus that deep internal attachment in which the screw is exposed to little or no load with an intimate contact between mating surfaces will result in good resistance to micromovement. This movement may be associated with crestal bone loss, as mentioned earlier [26]. In order to simplify the technique of placement of the abutments, an audible and tactile "click" feature was incorporated in the internal connection. Thus, the clinician will be able to tell when the abutment is in its intended position on the implant and the need for a radiograph following placement may be reduced. The internal connection when it is long enough may provide lateral stability for the restorative component from off-axis occlusal forces [25].

2.2. Types of abutments

Implant-supported restorations may be classified into two types according to the method by which they are attached to the implant: screw- and cement-retained implant restorations. Screw-retained implant restorations enable the direct attachment of the restoration to the implant or the abutment, whereas a cementing medium is used for the retention of the restoration onto the abutment for cement-retained implant restorations [25]. Comparison of the advantages and disadvantages of cement- and screw-retained techniques is shown in **Table 2** [27].

2.3. Abutment selection

For the single-tooth implant-supported restorations, an antirotational abutment mechanism is necessary. Currently, the most widely used mechanism is a hexagon with an internal connection. Because of the anatomical limitations related with the anterior single-tooth implant, the prosthetic abutment should be planned with an antirotational mechanism requiring a two-piece system. It may also be necessary to use angled abutment in order to compensate the implant insertion, which is not within the contours of the final restoration. This also forces the dentist to use at least two pieces: the abutment that engages the hexagon or antirotational design and an abutment screw that connects the abutment to the implant body [28]. Abutments are basically categorized into two types according to the fabrication technique:

- Prefabricated abutments
- Custom abutments

	Screw type	Cement type
Retrievability	Restorations can be removed/replaced without damage or the need for a new restoration	It is possible if weak cements were used, i.e., soft provisional cement, otherwise restorations have to be cut in order to remove them
Interocclusal space/ retention	It can also be used when the interocclusal space is limited, i.e., less than 4 mm	Minimum interocclusal space with minimum converges is needed to achieve an optimal retention
Limitation of mouth opening	The mouth opening should be enough for the use of different tools required for screwing and torquing the screws	A restricted mouth opening is less problematic than with the use of the screw-retained restorations
Occlusal loading	Unlikely to reduce the occlusal load on the restoration and the implant body	The use of soft provisional cement may reduce the occlusal load on the restoration and the implant body
Peri-implant inflammation	The adaptation between the restoration and the underlying implant is significantly better than that in the case of cement-retained counterpart	The difficulty of removing the cement and the inferiority of margin adaptation between the restoration and the abutment, when this margin is placed subgingivally can cause peri-implant soft tissue inflammation
Esthetics and occlusion	The implant needs to be placed in its optimal angulation in the anterior zone. The screw hole may interfere with the creation of an ideal occlusal morphology as well as with esthetics. The screw hole could weaken the porcelain veneer	Even if the implant angulation is not optimal, the restoration could still have good esthetics The ideal occlusal morphology can be created in the laboratory in the normal way as in the conventional restorations
Cost	The cost in terms of laboratory time and materials is much more than that for the cement-retained restorations	The materials and techniques used for the fabrication of the conventional restorations can be used in this situation

Table 2. Comparison of cement- and screw-retained restorations [27].

2.3.1. *Prefabricated abutments*

The prefabricated abutment is prepared by the manufacturer from different materials and provides a connection between the implant and the restoration, with different platform width, length, and gingival output profile. These abutments can be fabricated from titanium or its alloy, titanium with titanium nitride coating, or ceramic (alumina or zirconia) materials. They may also be angled or straight. The preangled abutment has varied angulations provided by manufacturers, usually 15 and 25 degrees off-axis (**Figure 2**) [29].

2.3.2. *Custom abutments*

The custom abutments are preferred for the esthetic and function in the anterior restorations. In the posterior region, it has been reported that the use of custom abutments is more successful than prefabricated abutments because of the small diameter implants due to insufficient bone mass, chewing forces in these regions are high and gingivae are wider [30].

Titanium abutments are considered as a 'gold standard' because of their clinical success rates and improved physical properties [31]. However, titanium abutments have been reported to cause reflection and grayish coloration of the mucosa around the implant [32]. Abutments made from full ceramics provide optimum esthetics when used in conjunction with full ceramic curtain restorations, reducing shading in soft tissue. Yttrium-stabilized tetragonal zirconia polycrystals (Y-TZPs) have begun to be used as abutment materials due to their durability and biocompatibility in implant-supported fixed dentures. Besides the esthetic qualities of zirconia abutments, they have a high corrosion resistance and a low plaque build-up [33, 34]. Tan et al. studied the zirconia's biocompatibility of abutments and did not encounter any complications that occurred in the soft tissue. Zirconia reported that less bacterial involvement occurred on the abutment surface than titanium [35].

Zirconia has been reported in abutments in the implanted platform, in the neck region of the connection, and in titanium abrasions and fractures [36–38]. It has been reported that the causes of wear and fracture may be due to differences in the hardness values of titanium and zirconia materials. Due to these observable complications, a system is created in which a zirconia abutment is made up of a titanium neck and a neck of the abutment-implant connection,

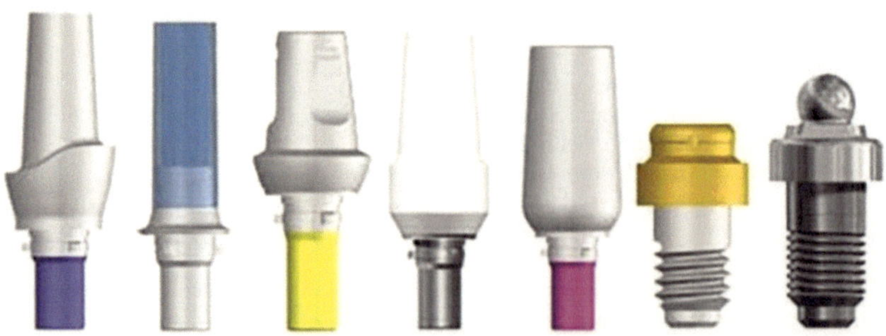

Figure 2. Different abutment types [29].

and this system is called a "hybrid abutment." With this system, the durability of titanium and the esthetic qualities of zirconia have been used together to become an alternative treatment for individual abutments [36, 37, 39]. With the understanding that the durability properties of hybrid abutments are higher than that of single-piece zirconia abutments, manufacturers have begun to produce titanium abutments in which they use as "ti-base" for use in accordance with existing implant sizes. Thus, the zirconia abutment on the titanium platform can be prepared and used in one piece, combined with the technique proposed by the firm [39].

Many companies that produce custom abutments for individuals can produce zirconia abutments in various color alternatives prepared beforehand by sintering in different color solutions or in different colors of zirconia blocks [40]. In recent years, monolithic zirconia onto ti-base, which is reported to have a high light transmission, has begun to be used as a hybrid abutment [41].

Different types of implant abutments have been described in the literature for use in the anterior region. The selection of an implant abutment in the anterior region is related to the factors: (1) smile line, (2) thickness of the peri-implant mucosa, (3) implant angulation, (4) restoration material, (5) interocclusal space, (6) type of the restoration related with the retention (screw- or cement-retained), (7) clinician's selection, and (8) cost of the treatment [22].

Patient's smile line can be categorized as low, medium, high, and gummy smile. When the smile line of the patient is low, there is no need to use esthetic abutment in no case. When the patient's smile line is from medium to gummy smile, selection of abutment material depends on the thickness of the buccal peri-implant mucosa. The abutment should be ceramic when the thickness of the buccal gingiva is ≤2 mm regardless of the bone thickness. When the buccal mucosa thickness exceeds 2 mm, there will be no esthetic problems due to titanium abutment use. Previous studies reported that 80% of the patients have buccal gingiva thickness less than 1.5 mm in the anterior region that means that zirconia abutment is necessary for most of the anterior restorations [42].

For anterior single-tooth implant-supported restorations, various options of abutments for cement retention are available:

1. A two-piece abutment for cement with minimal flare from the implant body
2. A two-piece abutment wider than the implant body
3. A two-piece anatomical abutment similar in shape to the cross section of a tooth
4. A plastic castable UCLA-type coping
5. UCLA-type machined/plastic cast to cylinder and abutment screw
6. Ceramic
7. Preangled abutment fabricated by the manufacturers with different angulations, usually with 15 and 25 degrees [43].

Manufacturers usually prefer the fabrication of the abutments wider than the implant body. An abutment with a wider cervical region enables obtaining an emergence profile for the crown, ensures a greater retention area, and provides a greater premade taper of the abutment. The dentist can customize the abutment preparation, condition, and site for each patient. In addition, the wider abutment and chamfer margin facilitate cement retrieval in subgingival margin applications. This is the most popular abutment used for the direct intraoral technique. The accuracy of the machined implant-abutment interface makes it a popular option. However, the wider abutment design has some disadvantages [29]:

1. The wider abutment is wider all around the implant body. When too close to the adjacent tooth/implant, too buccal, or too lingual, the abutment must be prepared further.
2. The wider abutment creates an undercut where it tapers down to the implant body, with several inherent problems. The crown margin must be placed above the undercut. If the undercut is more than 1 or 2 mm, long-term soft tissue shrinkage is likely to expose a metal band below the crown margin resulting in compromised esthetics.
3. If the implant was placed below the crestal bone, the restoring dentist cannot set the abutment on the implant platform without an osteoplasty around the implant, unless Stage I healing screw was of the same dimension as the wider abutment (in which case the osteoplasty would have been performed by the surgeon at implant insertion) [29].

The anatomical abutments (custom-made or premade) present similar advantages and disadvantages as the wider abutment posts. One more advantage is that because anterior teeth are wider faciolingually than mesiodistally, the abutment can reflect the natural tooth cross section [29].

An abutment with minimum flare presents several advantages:

- One size of abutment may be used for most of the patients.
- The abutment is seated on the implant platform and engages the hexagon without circumferential hard or soft tissue interference, which is beneficial because the abutment-to-implant connection may be several millimeters below the tissue.
- Minimal preparation is required if the implant is not in ideal position.
- The emergence profile of the crown is used to create the gingival contour and may be customized to the specific requirement of each area.
- The margin of the crown may be a knife-edge, chamfer, or shoulder and may be placed anywhere on the abutment.
- A knife-edge margin may be extended or shortened in the laboratory once the tissue model is fabricated.
- The abutment can be used for direct and indirect crown fabrication techniques [29].

The disadvantages of an abutment of similar diameter as the implant crest module include (1) a less tapered abutment, (2) a thinner outer wall of the abutment, (3) less material to prepare when a chamfer or a shoulder margin is preferred, and (4) no clear marking for the laboratory to determine the desired margin location unless a small chamfer is present on the selected abutment [29].

2.3.2.1. *Clinical cases*

Case 1: The extraoral picture taken from a patient with an osseointegrated implant on the left upper lateral region can be seen in **Figure 3**. Temporary screw-retained crown restoration was prepared and checked for approximately 3 months in order to obtain the recontouring of the emergence profile and interproximal papilla (**Figure 4**). Optimal emergence profile and soft tissue contouring achieved before fabrication of the final restoration can be seen in **Figure 5**. In **Figure 6**, the final crown restoration applied onto custom abutment, which was screw-retained 7 months after the implant surgery can be seen with satisfactory recontoured peri-implanter soft tissue and interproximal papilla. When the distance from the contact point of the crowns to the crest of bone is ≤5 mm, there will be no need for periodontal surgery in order to obtain the interproximal dental papilla (**Figure 7**) [44].

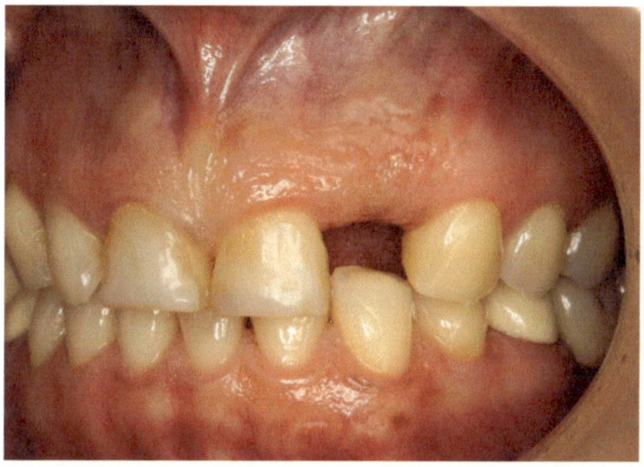

Figure 3. Soft tissue (4 months after implant surgery).

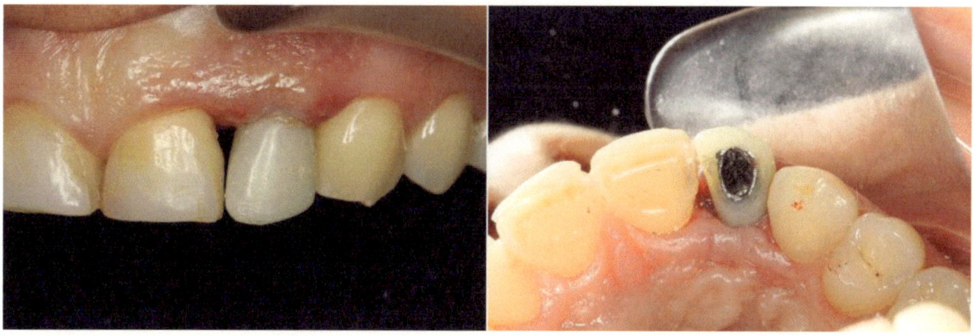

Figure 4. Buccal and palatinal view of screw-retained temporary acrylic crown prepared on prefabricated titanium abutment (4 months after implant surgery).

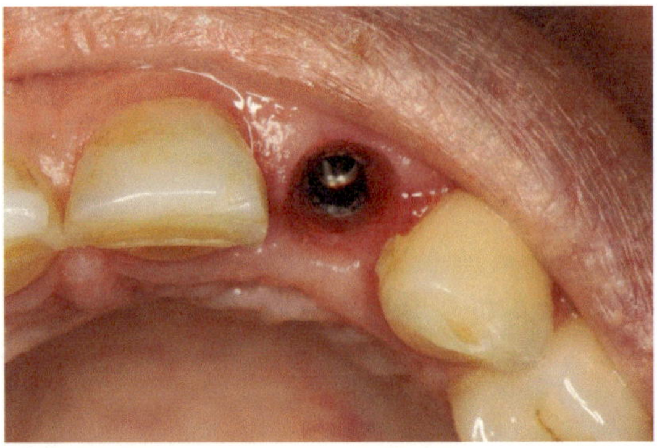

Figure 5. Reshaped emergence profile of the upper lateral incisor tooth.

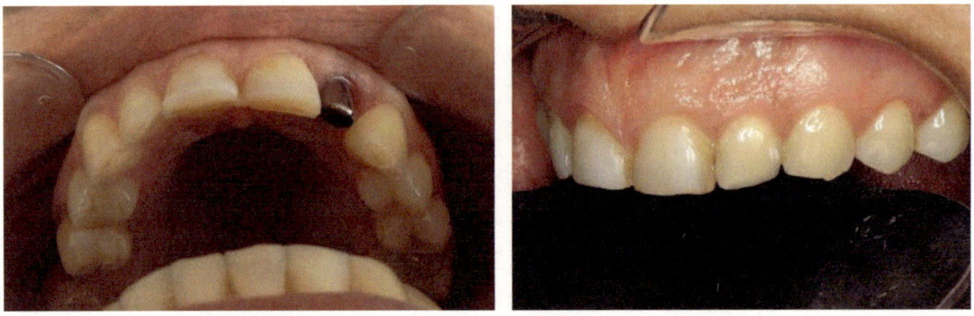

Figure 6. Final crown prepared on custom abutment by the application of veneering porcelain directly on titanium substructure (7 months after implant surgery).

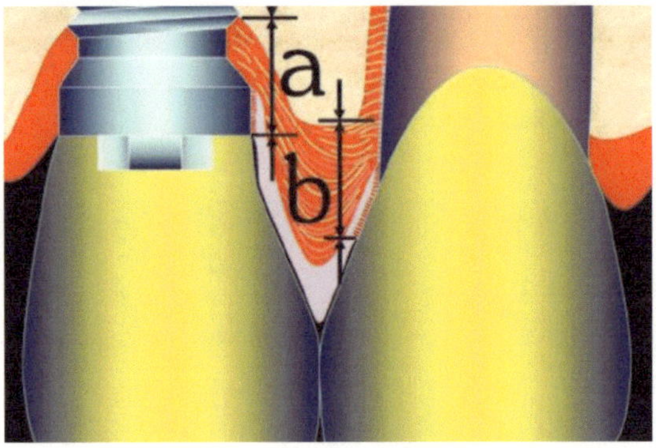

Figure 7. Schematic diagram showing the distance from the contact point of the crowns to the crest of bone.

Case 2: The extraoral picture taken from a patient with an osseointegrated implant on the left upper central incisor region can be seen in **Figures 8** and **9**. Temporary screw-retained crown restoration was prepared and checked for approximately 3 months in order to obtain the recontouring of the emergence profile and interproximal papilla (**Figures 8** and **9**). Following

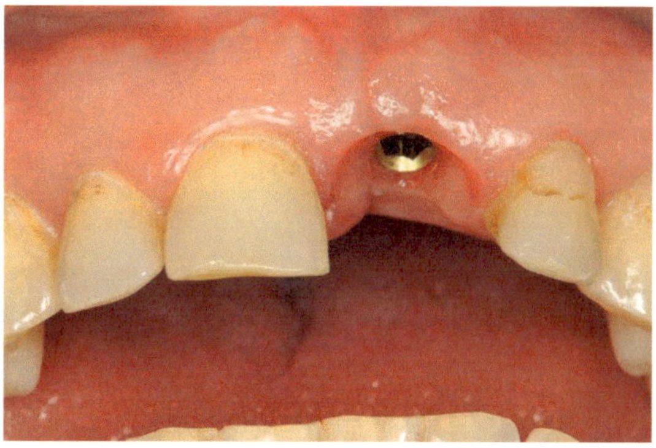

Figure 8. Reshaped emergence profile of the upper left central incisor tooth from buccal view.

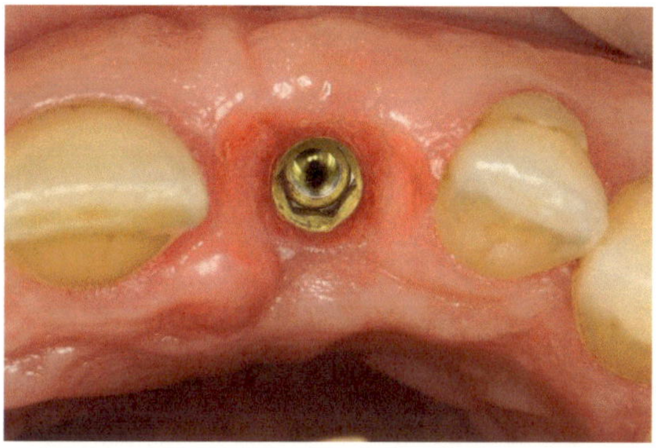

Figure 9. Reshaped emergence profile of upper left central incisor tooth from occlusal view.

the impression of the implant site, custom abutment design was achieved with the aid of a special CAD/CAM software (**Figures 10–12**). In **Figure 13**, custom designed hybrid abutment can be seen following the milling. Following the intraoral check of the custom abutment (**Figure 14**), the feldspathic layering porcelain was applied directly onto the hybrid abutment (**Figure 15**). In **Figures 16** and **17**, the final crown restoration applied onto the custom abutment, which was screw-retained 7 months after the implant surgery can be seen with satisfactory recontoured peri-implanter soft tissue and interproximal papilla.

2.4. Comparison of fracture strength of prefabricated and custom abutments

Most of the studies evaluating the custom abutments in the literature are in-vitro and short-term clinical follow-ups [45–58]. In-vitro studies showed that zirconia-based custom abutments have almost two times higher fracture strength than the alumina-based ones [45, 51]. Although zirconia-based abutments have lower fracture strength than titanium abutments, they were reported to be appropriate for use in clinical practice because of having two times higher strength than biting forces [45, 51]. A recent study reported that fracture strength of custom abutments was higher than prefabricated abutments, which were fabricated with the

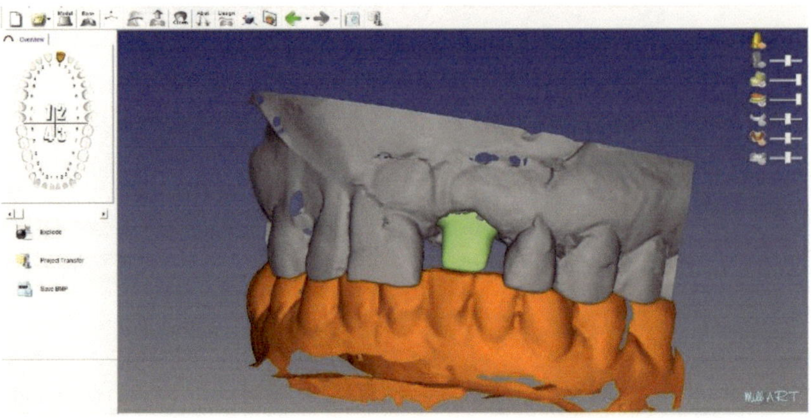

Figure 10. Designing the form of the hybrid abutment according to the occlusion with a CAD/CAM software.

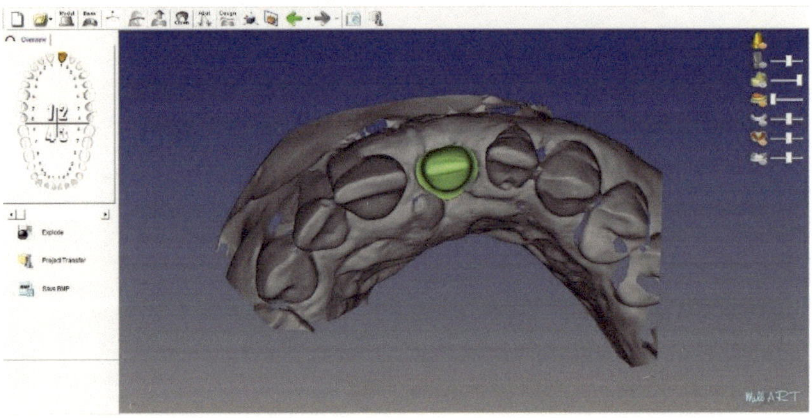

Figure 11. Occlusal view of the designed custom abutment.

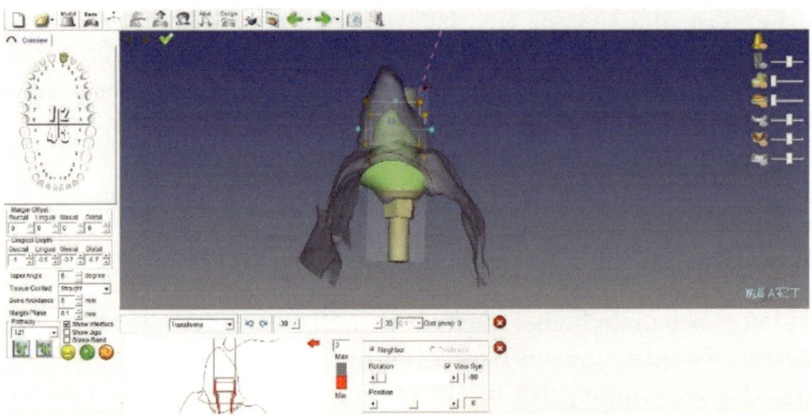

Figure 12. Sectional view of titanium and zirconia parts of the custom designed hybrid abutment.

http://dx.doi.org/10.5772/intechopen.80965

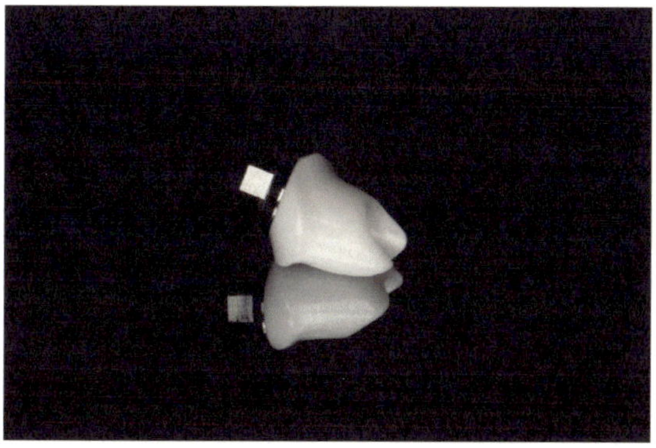

Figure 13. Designed hybrid abutment following milling with a CAM machine.

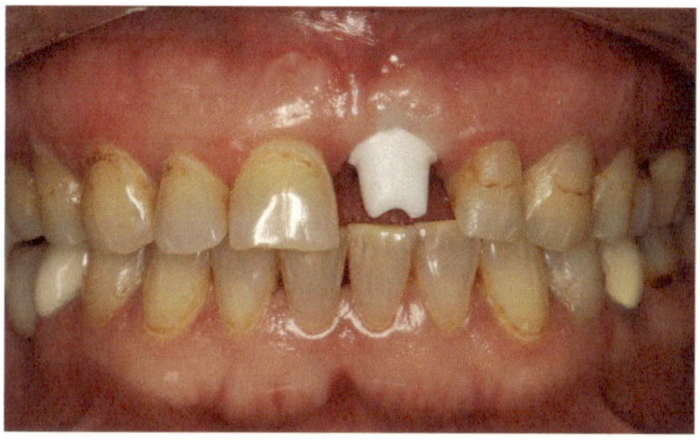

Figure 14. Intraoral check of the abutment.

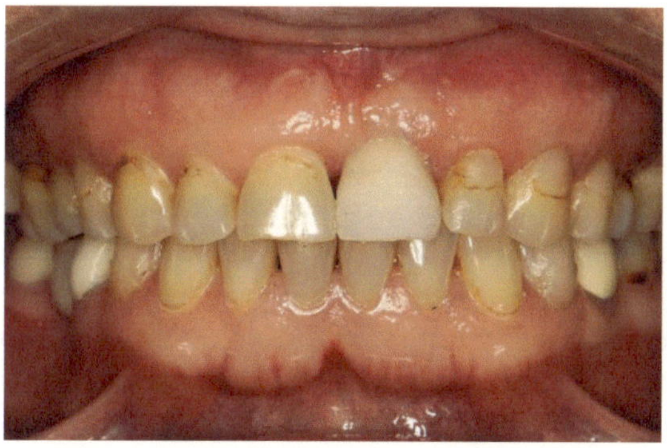

Figure 15. Dentin try-in of screw-retained monolithic implant-supported crown.

same CAD/CAM system [52]. Zembic et al. evaluated titanium- and zirconia-based custom abutments for the anterior single-tooth implant restorations and reported that biological and technical complication rates for both groups were similar at the end of 5 years usage [50]. Vanlıoğlu et al. compared prefabricated titanium and custom hybrid abutments applied onto

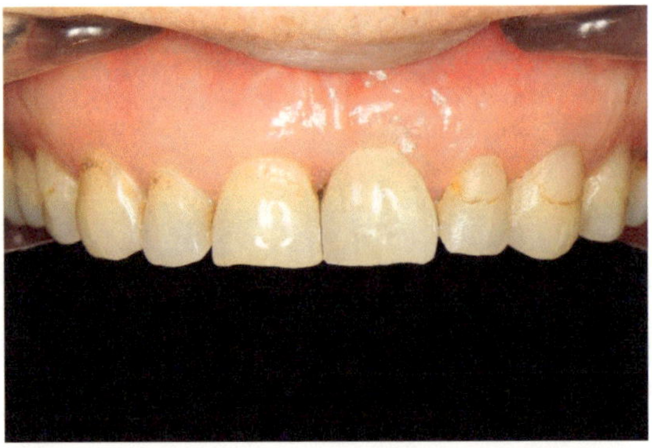

Figure 16. Screw-retained monolithic implant-supported crown.

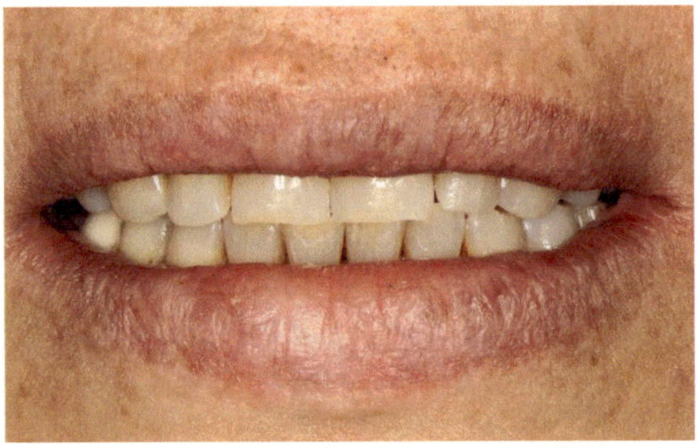

Figure 17. Labial view of the implant-supported crown.

narrow-diameter implants and reported a 100% survival rate at the end of 5 years follow-up [55]. The authors argue that hybrid abutments can be safely used for narrow-diameter implants as well as implants with standard diameters [55]. Prefabricated zirconia-based abutments showed significantly higher fracture strength than the zirconia-based abutments prepared by milling in the laboratory [46]. In-vitro studies showed that for the prefabricated abutments with zirconia neck, fracture occurs mostly at the neck region with varying rates for both the implants with internal and external connections [46]. A study comparing the fracture strength of prefabricated and hybrid abutments applied onto internal and external connected implants revealed that hybrid abutments with internal connection showed significantly higher strength than prefabricated abutments with internal and external connections [58]. Thulasidas et al. compared the fracture strength of angled prefabricated zirconia and custom hybrid abutments and reported that hybrid abutments showed higher strength than angled prefabricated abutments, and both groups showed lower strength values following artificial aging [53]. Similarly, another study evaluating anterior single-tooth restorations revealed that hybrid abutments prepared with 20° angle showed higher strength than straight prefabricated abutments [54]. It was also reported that fractures occurred mostly at implant-abutment interface [54].

3. Conclusions

Custom abutments designed individually with CAD/CAM systems provide optimal esthetics and function while preventing the technician to make possible mistakes during fabrication. In the future, developments in implant dentistry may enable fabrication of stronger abutments in less time and cost, and this will make it possible for the clinicians to make more satisfactory restorations with higher survival rates. Recent studies evaluating the fracture strength of custom and prefabricated abutments mostly report that custom abutments have several advantages and superiority compared to prefabricated ones. However, in-vitro study results related with custom abutment usage must be definitely supported with various long-term clinical follow-up studies in near future before recommending to the clinicians.

Author details

Pinar Turkoglu[1]*, Adnan Kose[2] and Deniz Sen[1]

*Address all correspondence to: drpturkoglu@yahoo.com

1 Department of Prosthodontics, Faculty of Dentistry, Istanbul University, Istanbul, Turkey

2 Private Practice, Istanbul, Turkey

References

[1] Jemt T. Modified single and short span restorations supported by osseointegrated fixtures in the partially edentulous jaw. The Journal of Prosthetic Dentistry. 1986;**55**:243-246. DOI: 10.1016/0022-3913(86)90352-5

[2] Avivi-Arber L, Zarb GA. Clinical effectiveness of implant-supported single-tooth replacement: The Toronto study. The International Journal of Oral & Maxillofacial Implants. 1996;**11**:311-321

[3] Lewis S, Beumer J, Hornburg W, Moy P. The "UCLA" abutment. The International Journal of Oral & Maxillofacial Implants. 1988;**3**:183-189

[4] Pjetursson BE, Tan K, Lang NP, Bragger U, Egger M, Zwahlen M. A systematic review of the survival and complication rates of fixed partial dentures (FPDs) after an observation period of at least 5 years. Clinical Oral Implants Research. 2004;**15**:625-642. DOI: 10.1111/j.1600-0501.2004.01120.x

[5] Andersson B. Implants for single-tooth replacement. A clinical and experimental study on the Branemark CeraOne system. Swedish Dental Journal. Supplement. 1995;**108**:1-41

[6] Sailer I, Philipp A, Zembic A, Pjetursson BE, Hammerle CH, Zwahlen M. A systematic review of the performance of ceramic and metal implant abutments supporting fixed

implant reconstructions. Clinical Oral Implants Research. 2009;**20**(suppl 4):4-31. DOI: 10.1111/j.1600-0501.2009.01787.

[7] Zembic A, Sailer I, Jung RE, Hammerle CH. Randomized-controlled clinical trial of customized zirconia and titanium implant abutments for single-tooth implants in canine and posterior regions: 3-year results. Clinical Oral Implants Research. 2009;**20**:802-808. DOI: 10.1111/j.1600-0501.2009.01717.x

[8] Jung RE, Holderegger C, Sailer I, Khraisat A, Suter A, Hammerle CH. The effect of all-ceramic and porcelain-fused-to-metal restorations on marginal peri-implant soft tissue color: A randomized controlled clinical trial. The International Journal of Periodontics & Restorative Dentistry. 2008;**28**:357-365. DOI: 10.5167/uzh-9284

[9] Park SE, Da Silva JD, Weber HP, Ishika-wa-Nagai S. Optical phenomenon of peri-implant soft tissue. Part I. Spectrophotometric assessment of natural tooth gingiva and peri-implant mucosa. Clinical Oral Implants Research. 2007;**18**:569-574. DOI: 10.1111/j.1600-0501.2007.01391.x

[10] Bressan E, Paniz G, Lops D, Corazza B, Romeo E, Favero G. Influence of abutment material on the gingival color of implant-supported all-ceramic restorations: A prospective multicenter study. Clinical Oral Implants Research. 2011;**22**:631-637. DOI: 10.1111/j.1600-0501.2010.02008.x

[11] van Brakel R, Noordmans HJ, Frenken J, de Roode R, de Wit GC, Cune MS. The effect of zirconia and titanium implant abutments on light reflection of the supporting soft tissues. Clinical Oral Implants Research. 2011;**22**:1172-1178. DOI: 0.1111/j.1600-0501.2010.02082.x

[12] Prestipino V, Ingber A. Esthetic high strength implant abutments. Part I. Journal of Esthetic Dentistry. 1993;**5**:29-36. DOI: 10.1111/j.1708-8240.1993.tb00741.x

[13] Prestipino V, Ingber A. Esthetic high strength implant abutments. Part II. Journal of Esthetic Dentistry. 1993;**5**:63-68. DOI: 10.1111/j.1708-8240.1993.tb00750.x

[14] Prestipino V, Ingber A. All-ceramic implant abutments. Esthetic indications. Journal of Esthetic Dentistry. 1996;**8**:255-262. DOI: 10.1111/j.1708-8240.1996.tb00876.x

[15] Henriksson K, Jemt T. Evaluation of custom-made procera ceramic abutments for single-implant tooth replacement: A prospective 1-year follow-up study. The International Journal of Prosthodontics. 2003;**16**:626-630

[16] Glauser R, Sailer I, Wohlwend A, et al. Experimental zirconia abutments for implant-supported single-tooth restorations in esthetically demanding regions: 4-year results of a prospective clinical study. The International Journal of Prosthodontics. 2004;**17**:285-290

[17] Scarano A, Piattelli M, Caputi S, Favero GA, Piattelli A. Bacterial adhesion on commercially pure titanium and zirconium oxide disks: An in vivo human study. Journal of Periodontology. 2004;**75**:292-296

[18] Ichikawa Y, Akagawa Y, Nikai H, Tsuru H. Tissue compatibility and stability of a new zirconia ceramic in vivo. The Journal of Prosthetic Dentistry. 1992;**68**:322-326

[19] Piconi C, Maccauro G. Zirconia as a ceramic biomaterial. Biomaterials. 1999;**20**:1-25

[20] Marchack CB. A custom titanium abutment for the anterior single-tooth implant. Journal of Prosthetic Dentistry. 1996;**76**:288-291

[21] Ekfeldt A, Fürst B, Carlsson GE. Zirconia abutments for single-tooth implant restorations: A retrospective and clinical follow-up study. Clinical Oral Implants Research. 2011; **22**(11):1308-1314

[22] Bidra AS, Rungruanganunt P. Clinical outcomes of implant abutments in the anterior region: A systematic review. Journal of Esthetic and Restorative Dentistry. 2013;**25**(3): 159-176

[23] Garner LD, Kotwal NS. Correlation study of incisive biting forces with age, sex, and anterior occlusion. Journal of Dental Research. 1973;**52**:698-702

[24] Kumagai H, Suzuki T, Hamada T, et al. Occlusal force distribution on the dental arch during various levels of clenching. Journal of Oral Rehabilitation. 1999;**26**:932-935

[25] Warreth A et al. An introduction to single implant abutments. Dental Update. 2013;**40**(1):7-17

[26] Hermann JS, Schoolfield JD, Schenk RK, Buser D, Cochran DL. Influence of the size of the microgap on crestal bone changes around titanium implants. A histometric evaluation of unloaded non-submerged implants in the canine mandible. Journal of Periodontology. 2001;**72**:1372-1383

[27] Newsome P, Reaney D, Owen S. Screw-versus cement-retained crowns. Irish Dentist. 2011;**3**:22-25

[28] Kallus T et al. Clinical evaluation of angulated abutments for the Brånemark system: A pilot study. International Journal of Oral & Maxillofacial Implants. 1990;**5**:1

[29] Misch CE. Dental Implant Prosthetics-E-Book. St.Louis: Elsevier, Mosby; 2014

[30] Joda T, Wittneben JG, Brägger U. Digital implant impressions with the "Individualized Scanbody Technique" for emergence profile support. Clinical Oral Implants Research. 2014;**25**:395-397

[31] Osman RB, Swain VB. A critical review of dental implant materials with an emphasis on titanium versus zirconia. Materials. 2015;**8**:932-958

[32] Ormianer Z, Schiroli G. Maxillary single-tooth replacement utilizing a novel ceramic restorative system: Results to 30 months. The Journal of Oral Implantology. 2006;**32**:190-199

[33] Firidinoğlu K, Toksavul S, Toman M. İmplant destekli sabit protezlerde seramik abutment kullanımı. Ege Üniversitesi Dişhekimliği Fakültesi Dergisi. 2007;**28**:145-150

[34] Butz F, Heydecke G, Okutan M, Strub JR. Survival rate, fracture strength and failure mode of ceramic implant abutments after chewing simulation. Journal of Oral Rehabilitation. 2005;**32**:838-843

[35] Tan PL, Dunne JT. An esthetic comparison of a metal ceramic crown and cast metal abutment with an all-ceramic crown and zirconia abutment: A clinical report. The Journal of Prosthetic Dentistry. 2004;**91**(3):215-218

[36] Binon PP. Implants and components: Entering the new millennium. The International Journal of Oral & Maxillofacial Implants. 2000;**15**:76-94

[37] Brodbeck U. The ZiReal Post: A new ceramic implant abutment. Journal of Esthetic and Restorative Dentistry. 2003;**15**:10-23

[38] Stimmelmayr M, Edelhoff D, Guth JF, Erdelt K, Happe A, Beuer F. Wear at the titanium-titanium and the titanium-zirconia implant-abutment interface: A comparative in vitro study. Dental Materials. 2012;**28**:1215-1220

[39] Kurbad A, Kurbad S. CAD/CAM-based implant abutments. International Journal of Computerized Dentistry. 2013;**16**(2):125-141

[40] Gehrke P, Johannson D, Fischer C, Stawarczyk B, Beuer F. In vitro fatigue and fracture resistance of one- and two-piece CAD/CAM zirconia implant abutments. The International Journal of Oral & Maxillofacial Implants. 2015;**30**(3):546-554

[41] Martinez-Rus F, Ferreiroa A, Ozcan M, Bartolome JF, Pradies G. Fracture resistance of crowns cemented on titanium and zirconia implant abutments: A comparison of monolithic versus manually veneered all-ceramic systems. The International Journal of Oral & Maxillofacial Implants. 2012;**27**:1448-1455

[42] Jung RE, Sailer I, Hämmerle CH, Attin T, Schmidlin P. In vitro color changes of soft tissues caused by restorative materials. The International Journal of Periodontics & Restorative Dentistry. 2007;**27**(3):251-257

[43] Daftary F, Bahat O. Prosthetically formulated natural aesthetics in implant prostheses. Practical Periodontics and Aesthetic Dentistry: Ppad 6. 1994;**9**:75-83

[44] Tarnow DP, Magner AW, Fletcher P. The effect of the distance from the contact point to the crest of bone on the presence or absence of the interproximal dental papilla. Journal of Periodontology. 1992;**63**(12):995-996

[45] Yildirim M, Fischer H, Marx R, Edelhoff D. In vivo fracture resistance of implant-supported all-ceramic restorations. The Journal of Prosthetic Dentistry. 2003;**90**(4):325-331

[46] Alqahtani F, Flinton R. Postfatigue fracture resistance of modified prefabricated zirconia implant abutments. The Journal of Prosthetic Dentistry. 2014;**112**(2):299-305

[47] Manicone PF, Rossi Iommetti P, Raffaelli L. An overview of zirconia ceramics: Basic properties and clinical applications. Journal of Dentistry. 2007;**35**(11):819-826

[48] Ozkurt Z, Kazazoğlu E. Clinical success of zirconia in dental applications. Journal of Prosthodontics. 2010;**19**:64-68

[49] Ardlin BI. Transformation-thoughened zirconia for dental inlays, crowns and bridges: Chemical stability and effect of low temperature aging on the flexural strength and surface structure. Dental Materials. 2002;**18**(8):590-595

[50] Zembic A, Bösch A, Jung RE, Hämmerle CH, Sailer I. Five-year results of a randomized controlled clinical trial comparing zirconia and titanium abutments supporting single implant crowns in canine and posterior regions. Clinical Oral Implants Research. 2013;**24**(4):384-390

[51] Mitsias ME, Silva NR, Pines M, Stappert C, Thompson VP. Reliability and fatigue damage modes of zirconia and titanium abutments. The International Journal of Prosthodontics. 2010;**23**(1):56-59

[52] Park JI, Lee Y, Lee JH, Kim YL, Bae JM, Cho HW. Comparison of fracture resistance and fit accuracy of customized zirconia abutments with prefabricated zirconia abutments in internal hexagonal implants. Clinical Implant Dentistry and Related Research. 2013;**15**(5):769-778

[53] Thulasidas S, Givan DA, Lemons JE, O'Neal SJ, Ramp LC, Liu PR. Influence of implant angulation on the fracture resistance of zirconia abutments. Journal of Prosthodontics. 2015;**24**(2):127-135

[54] Nothdurft FP, Doppler KE, Erdelt KJ, Knauber AW, Pospiech PR. Fracture behavior of straight or angulated zirconia implant abutments supporting anterior single crowns. Clinical Oral Investigations. 2011;**15**(2):157-163

[55] Vanlıoglu BA, Özkan Y, Evren B, Özkan YK. Experimental custom-made zirconia abutments for narrow implants in esthetically demanding regions: A 5-year follow-up. The International Journal of Oral & Maxillofacial Implants. 2012;**27**(5):1239-1242

[56] Moon IS, Berglundh T, Abrahamsson I, Linder E, Lindhe J. The barrier between the keratinized mucosa and the dental implant. An experimental study in the dog. Journal of Clinical Periodontology. 1999;**26**(10):658-663

[57] Nascimento C, Pita MS, Pedrazzi V, de Albuquerque Junior RF, Ribeiro RF. In vivo evaluation of Candida spp. adhesion on titanium or zirconia abutment surfaces. Archives of Oral Biology. 2013;**58**(7):853-861

[58] Sailer I, Sailer T, Stawarczyk B, Jung RE, Hämmerle CH. In vitro study of the influence of the type of connection on the fracture load of zirconia abutments with internal and external implant-abutment connections. The International Journal of Oral & Maxillofacial Implants. 2009;**24**(5):850-858

Chapter 5

Peri-implantitis Microbiota

Dalia Khalil and Margareta Hultin

Additional information is available at the end of the chapter

http://dx.doi.org/10.5772/intechopen.79486

Abstract

Dental implant surgery has been a successful therapeutic option for the rehabilitation of partially or completely edentulous jaws for many years. However, evidence regarding the causative factors of peri-implant disease is still lacking. Peri-implantitis is an inflammatory disease affecting the soft and hard tissues surrounding osseointegrated implant associated with the formation of a bacterial biofilm on the implant surface close to the marginal tissues. The aim of this chapter is to summarize the knowledge regarding the microbiota associated with peri-implant infection and to review the different microbial diagnostic tests to understand the peri-implant microbiota, as well as summarize the present knowledge regarding management of peri-implantitis and propose further recommendations for future studies. This chapter shows that the scientific data regarding the microbiota responsible for peri-implantitis initiation and progression are still inconclusive. A microbiological test may thus be one diagnostic method to be used to understand the complexity of microbiota associated with the peri-implant sulcus. However, in order to resolve inflammation and arrest disease progression, the understanding of the biofilm development is essential.

Keywords: dental implant, peri-implant infection, peri-implantitis, peri-implant microbiota, peri-implant microbial test

1. Introduction

Dental implants have become a successful therapeutic option to replace missing tooth. It has been estimated that approximately 12 million implants are placed every year, worldwide [1]. With the global increase of dental implant placement, there is a continued need for investigation regarding the etiology, risk factors and treatment for dental implant complications. Moreover, the widespread use of dental implants has led to an increase in biofilm-mediated peri-implant disease. There is an undisputed effect between the formation of an oral biofilm on the implant surface and the initiation of the inflammatory process around osseointegrated dental implants [2].

Initially, clinical measures such as probing were not recommended since it was believed that this could harm the mucosal seal. Therefore, diagnostic measures were limited to the radiographic examination. Thus, disease remained undiagnosed for many years. Therefore, failing dental implants were not diagnosed, and only failed implants were detected where the implant needed to be removed [3]. First, the term peri-implantoclasia was used to describe the disease condition, that is, catabolic condition with/without sepsis or suppuration, around the dental implant [4, 5]. However, this term was replaced shortly after with *peri-implantitis*, which became the accepted terminology for the infectious nature of the pathologic condition surrounding peri-implant tissue [6, 7].

Peri-implantitis has been described as a "site specific" condition or as an "inflammatory bacterial driven destruction of the implant supporting apparatus," which means that microorganisms play an important role in peri-implantitis [8, 9]. The prevalence of peri-implantitis shows a wide range (10-25%) in different study populations primarily due to the definition of peri-implantitis, i.e. the chosen cut-off level for registering marginal bone loss and the duration of the patient's follow-up [10, 11]. However, one of the major challenges in the treatment of peri-implantitis is the lack of effective treatments.

2. Periodontitis versus peri-implantitis

Peri-implantitis is defined as an inflammatory disease affecting the soft and hard tissues surrounding osseointegrated functioning implants, while periodontitis is defined as inflammation affecting the tissues around the teeth [12, 13]. Despite the similarities between peri-implantitis and periodontitis, they seem to differ in extent, composition and progression of lesions [14, 15]. Peri-implant disease is known to be multifactorial with risk factors identical to periodontitis, including poor oral hygiene, smoking, diabetes, and genetic factors [2, 16]. History, or current periodontitis status, increases the risk of peri-implantitis [2, 16–19]. However, there is a complex interaction between the development of periodontitis and peri-implantitis and the formation of bacterial biofilm [2, 16].

One of the major anatomical differences between periodontal and peri-implant tissue is the presence of a periodontal ligament around the tooth, while the implant is in an ankylosed state. Although there is extensive information regarding the histopathological characteristics of human periodontal lesions, only a few studies have evaluated peri-implantitis lesions in humans. Berglundh et al. concluded in a systematic review that critical histopathological differences exist between the two lesions [20]. For example, the apical extension of the inflammatory cell infiltrate was more pronounced in peri-implantitis lesions compared to that in periodontal lesions. In peri-implantitis, the inflammatory cell infiltrate was, in most cases, located apical of the pocket epithelium. In both types of lesions, the infiltrate was dominated by plasma cells and lymphocytes, but in peri-implantitis, the neutrophil granulocytes and macrophages occurred in larger proportions [20]. In a recent animal study on mice, where periodontitis and peri-implantitis lesions were experimentally induced by ligatures, a striking difference was observed on comparing the spontaneous healing after ligature removal. More bone was regained after ligature removal around teeth compared with that around implants in the peri-implantitis lesions. The intrinsic ability of the periodontal ligament to repair bone around teeth may thus be one of several key factors influencing treatment outcomes of peri-implantitis [21]. Moreover, soft tissues around teeth and implants are of similar dimensions [3]. The outer surface of the gingiva and peri-implant mucosa is covered by keratinized oral epithelium, but the peri-implant mucosa continues marginally with a thin nonkeratinized barrier epithelium, which is similar to the junctional epithelium around teeth [3]. However, the reaction of the soft and hard tissue after microbial colonization is similar in many aspects [3].

It was previously believed that there are similarities between peri-implantitis and periodontitis microbiota, and that periodontal pathogens translocate into peri-implant tissue. These similarities were once considered a critical factor in disease causation [19]. Recently, it has been reported that peri-implantitis and periodontitis microbial environments are distinct, with differences in core microbiota between the two conditions [20, 22–24].

3. Peri-implant microbiology

Implant insertion appears to stimulate the mechanism of mature biofilm development. However, this initially formed biofilm is in a commensal state [25, 26]. The biofilm that surrounds healthy implants is confined supramucosally, regardless of the fact that it can be found in massive amounts [27]. Bacterial colonization starts approximately 30 min after the implant is inserted into the oral environment [28, 29]. Recently, studies identified more than 700 bacterial species and 25,000 phylotypes in the oral cavity [22, 30–32].

The bacterial composition of the peri-implant biofilm harbors a similar microbiota to that of the neighboring teeth [33], which means that teeth serve as reservoirs for bacterial colonization in the biofilm surrounding implants [6, 34–36]. Similarities between peri-implant and periodontal microflora have been shown in several studies [37–39]. The subgingival microbiota of diseased implants has generally been considered to share some common characteristics [33].

The peri-implant microbiota of healthy sites has been shown in some studies to be more diverse and complex than in peri-implantitis, which indicates that healthy sites have a more stable and healthy ecosystem [40, 41]. On the other hand, other studies have shown higher microbiota diversity in diseased subjects [42]. These observations demonstrate that the microbial communities in both healthy and diseased tissue are quite different; however, generally, most taxa are present in both conditions [42, 43].

The subgingival microbiota of healthy implants and peri-implantitis are colonized by periodontopathic microorganisms [44, 45]. For example, the peri-implantitis microbiota showed up to a 40% higher frequency of red complex and orange complex compared to healthy implants [8, 44, 46–51]. The most frequent periodontal pathogens presented in a peri-implantitis lesions are from genera such as Bacteroides, Prevotella, Porphyromonas, Treponema, and Tannerella [46, 52–54]. Moreover, there is an increase in the diversity of species in the more advanced stages of disease [51]. Previous studies suggest that periodontopathic bacteria are not the only periodontal pathogens active in peri-implantitis, and that noncultivable microorganisms such as asaccharolytic anaerobic Gram-positive rods **(AAGPRs)** and oxidized graphene nanoribbons **(OGNRs)** may also play an important role in peri-implantitis lesions [41, 44, 54–57]. In addition, Gram-negative microorganisms such as *Aggregatibacter actinomycetemcomitans* (Aa), *Parvimonas micra* (Pm), and *Campylobacter rectus* (Cr) were identified in 52% of the studies [46, 48, 58–65] presented in a systematic review by Lafaurie [44]. Few studies have shown the presence of *Pseudomonas aeruginosa, Candida albicans, Staphylococcus aureus,* and *Staphylococcus Warneri* in peri-implantitis lesions [46, 47, 66]. In addition, the Epstein-Barr virus has been considered an enhanced risk factor in peri-implantitis lesions [67, 68]. However, it is not yet considered a microbiologic marker for peri-implantitis [67, 68]. The role of phylum Synergistetes in peri-implantitis lesions is still debated. Some recent studies have shown a strong association between this phylum and the occurrence of peri-implantitis [69, 70], while others conclude there is no relationship [71]. Therefore, peri-implantitis lesions represent a heterogeneous infection [44].

There are many factors that determine the variation in peri-implant microbiota and also the degree of its shift from the healthy microbiota found in the peri-implant sulcus. These factors include differences in the microbiological detection methods used in various studies [45, 72]. Moreover, inter-individual variations in oral microbiota (such as the presence of pathologic conditions in the oral environment, for example, untreated periodontal disease, smokers, or the status of edentulous), study design (longitudinal or cross-sectional, number of participants), and how the samples are handled all influence variations between studies [14, 72, 73]. To date, there is still limited data on which bacteria are involved in the initiation and progression of peri-implantitis disease [15]. Therefore, we should emphasize the fact that regardless of the statistically significant changes in peri-implant microbiota, microbiome composition shows a high tendency for changes that lead to a shift from a healthy status to a diseased status [72].

4. Microbial diagnostic tests

To date, clinical and radiographic data are the main diagnostic methods for the diagnosis of peri-implant disease. However, these methods are limited because they only detect the disease after a certain level of destruction [45]. Therefore, the use of microbiological tests is important to be able to determine the microbiota associated with the peri-implant sulcus [45]. There are different ways of testing the bacterial composition at the peri-implant sites. First, the sample is collected using sterile paper points, a sterile periodontal probe or a curette. These samples are then analyzed either by culture-based methods, molecular methods, sequencing methods, or other advanced new methods (i.e., metagenomics).

Culture-based methods were the first approach in helping understanding the human microbiomes. However, 20–60% of the microbiome is known to be uncultivable [74]. The limitation of this technique is that it is both time-consuming, and the results underestimate the diversity of the human microbiota.

The molecular methods, such as PCR or DNA-DNA hybridization, help to increase the number of bacterial species known to be oral commensals, which leads to increased understanding of the disease process. These methods are faster and more sensitive than the culture-based ones, but are also limited because of the need to pre-select DNA probes for the specific bacterial taxa to be investigated [39]. Therefore, one has to be cautious when interpreting these results, as finding "unexpected" microbiota is impossible with these techniques, thus creating a risk of bias. However, these techniques have overcome the limitations of culturing techniques.

During the last few years, sequencing methods such as 16S rRNA have allowed the evaluation of an entire community's microbiome [39, 57]. These methods use a universal primer system to detect a broad range of bacterial taxa [75, 76] and discover previously new undetected and uncultivable bacteria [41, 57, 70]. Sequencing methods are able to overcome the limitations of the above-mentioned methods. On the other hand, this technique also has limitations. For example, in determining differences at the strain level, some taxa may escape detection due to less effective primer binding or differential amplification [39, 72].

Recently, some studies have used metagenomic methods for investigating microbiomes. This method is based on extracting DNA directly from the sample without "looking for" a specific organism and can be randomly sequenced or functionally screened for activities of interest [77]. These methods have recently provided valuable insights into the pathogenesis of periodontitis and may allow a paradigm shift in the understanding of peri-implantitis disease. However, studies using this technique are still ongoing.

5. Management of peri-implantitis

To date, there is no clear evidence to indicate what the initiating factors for peri-implant disease are. However, microbial infections with bacteria and possibly yeasts and viruses play an important role in the disease process [16, 46, 78, 79]. Peri-implantitis is always considered an infectious disease with the need for antimicrobial treatment to empirically target specific putative bacteria [78, 80–87]. The primary treatment goals of peri-implantitis are to resolve inflammation and arrest disease progression. Surface decontamination is important to consider during treatment. There is no gold standard in the treatment of peri-implantitis. However, surgical access with the adjunctive use of different chemical detergents, air powder abrasive devises or lasers have been previously presented to achieve surface decontamination [88].

Data regarding the effect of systematic antibiotics on peri-implantitis lesions are lacking long-term outcomes. Although the effect of systemic antimicrobials agents in the surgical treatment of peri-implantitis is still limited [38], time and dosage have made the risk of antibiotic resistance development a reality [78, 89]. Using antimicrobial agents may risk developing bacterial resistance and the overgrowth of superinfecting microorganisms that are difficult to eradicate [78]. The development of opportunistic pathogens, such as *S. aureus* or EBV, may lead to a change in the normal symbiotic ecosystem to a dysbiotic ecosystem by affecting the local innate immune response. This, in turn, leads to overgrowth of superinfecting bacteria and yeast [90–93]. The development of antimicrobial resistance will escalate peri-implant disease in the coming years. Therefore, the need for microbial sampling and testing is mandatory in order to prevent the risk of superinfection. These tests will identify the presence of ongoing specific microbial challenges that are difficult to eliminate and allow disease to progress.

Moreover, strict supportive maintenance therapy should be considered to prevent disease recurrence and to keep ecological balance in the oral microbiota [94]. Therefore, the presence of antimicrobial agents that do not alter colonization resistance will lead to a decrease in the risk of development, spread and dissemination of resistant strains among patients [91].

6. Conclusion and future perspectives

Peri-implantitis is heterogeneous, polymicrobial infection where certain core microbiota may pose a significant role. Scientific evidence identifying the specific microbiota responsible for the development and progression of peri-implant infection is still inconclusive. A review of the literature points to an enrichment of well-recognized pathogens in addition to newly proposed pathogenic microorganisms, several of which have not yet been cultivated. Therefore, understanding the peri-implantitis microbiota will improve strategies for prevention, supportive therapy, risk assessment, early diagnosis of peri-implantitis, and timely intervention—all key aspects of long-term survival of dental implants [95]. Based on the available knowledge presented in the literature, **Figure 1** summarizes important tips to the clinician. Future studies designed to understand the peri-implantitis microbiota should include careful selection of cases and controls, and the incorporation of state-of-the-art approaches, such as metagenomics [95].

MESSAGE TO THE CLINICIAN

- Formation of an oral biofilm on the implant surface play an important role in peri-implantitis.
- Supportive maintenance therapy should always be included in the plan for long term maintenance of patients treated with dental implants to help keeping ecological balance in the oral microbiota
- Peri-implantitis lesions represent a heterogeneous infection with well-recognized pathogens in addition to newly proposed pathogenic microorganisms, several of which have not yet been cultivated.
- Clinical and radiographic examination for peri-implantitis are limited for early diagnosis and the use of microbiological tests can therefore be of great value.

Figure 1. Tips for the clinician regarding peri-implantitis.

Author details

Dalia Khalil[1,2*] and Margareta Hultin[2]

*Address all correspondence to: dalia.khalil@ki.se

1 Division of Periodontology, Implant Clinic, King Fahad General Hospital, Jeddah, Saudi Arabia

2 Department of Dental Medicine, Division of Periodontology, Karolinska Institutet, Huddinge, Sweden

References

[1] Albrektsson T, Dahlin C, Jemt T, Sennerby L, Turri A, Wennerberg A. Is marginal bone loss around oral implants the result of a provoked foreign body reaction? Clinical Implant Dentistry and Related Research. 2014;**16**(2):155-165

[2] Lindhe J, Meyle J, Group DoEWoP. Peri-implant diseases: Consensus report of the sixth European workshop on periodontology. Journal of Clinical Periodontology. 2008;**35** (8 Suppl):282-285

[3] Charalampakis G. Peri-Implantitis from a Microbiological Perspective. 2013

[4] Boucher CO. Current Clinical Dental Terminology, a Glossary of Accepted Terms in all Disciplines of Dentistry. St. Louis: Mosby; 1963

[5] Jermyn AC. Peri-implantoclaisa: Cause and treatment. International Journal of Implant Dentistry. 1958;**5**:25-48

[6] Mombelli A, Oosten M, Schürch E, Lang N. The microbiota associated with successful or failing osseointegrated titanium implants. Oral Microbiology and Immunology. 1987; **2**(4):145-151

[7] Levignac J. Periimplantation osteolysis- periimplantosis - periimplantitis. [Article in French]. Revue Française d'Odonto-Stomatologie 1965;**8**:1251-1260

[8] Mombelli A, van Oosten MAC, Schürch E, Lang NP. The microbiota associated with successful or failing osseointegrated titanium implants. Oral Microbiology and Immunology. 1987;**2**(4):145-151

[9] Tonetti M. Peri-implantitis: Biological considerations. Journal de Parodontologie. 1996; **15**:269-284

[10] Tomasi C, Derks J. Clinical research of peri-implant diseases--quality of reporting, case definitions and methods to study incidence, prevalence and risk factors of peri-implant diseases. Journal of Clinical Periodontology. 2012;**39**(12 Suppl):207-223

[11] Mombelli A, Muller N, Cionca N. The epidemiology of peri-implantitis. Clinical Oral Implants Research. 2012;**23**(Suppl 6):67-76

[12] Zarb GAAT. Consensus report: Towards optimized treatment outcomes for dental implants. The Journal of Prosthetic Dentistry. 1998;**80**(6):641

[13] Zitzmann NU, Berglundh T. Definition and prevalence of peri-implant diseases. Journal of Clinical Periodontology. 2008;**35**(8 Suppl):286-291

[14] Lang NP, Berglundh T. Periimplant diseases: Where are we now?--consensus of the seventh European workshop on periodontology. Journal of Clinical Periodontology. 2011; **11**:178-181

[15] Becker ST, Beck-Broichsitter BE, Graetz C, Dorfer CE, Wiltfang J, Hasler R. Peri-implantitis versus periodontitis: Functional differences indicated by transcriptome profiling. Clinical Implant Dentistry and Related Research. 2014;**16**(3):401-411

[16] Heitz-Mayfield LJA, Lang NP. Comparative biology of chronic and aggressive periodontitis vs. peri-implantitis. Periodontology 2000. 2010;**53**(1):167-181

[17] Karoussis IK, Salvi GE, Heitz-Mayfield LJA, Brägger U, Hämmerle CHF, Lang NP. Long-term implant prognosis in patients with and without a history of chronic periodontitis: A 10-year prospective cohort study of the ITI® dental implant system. Clinical Oral Implants Research. 2003;**14**(3):329-339

[18] Roos-Jansaker AM, Lindahl C, Renvert H, Renvert S. Nine- to fourteen-year follow-up of implant treatment. Part II: Presence of peri-implant lesions. Journal of Clinical Periodontology. 2006;**33**(4):290-295

[19] Heitz-Mayfield LJ. Peri-implant diseases: Diagnosis and risk indicators. Journal of Clinical Periodontology. 2008;**35**(8 Suppl):292-304

[20] Berglundh T, Zitzmann NU, Donati M. Are peri-implantitis lesions different from periodontitis lesions?, Journal of Clinical Periodontology. 2011;**38**(11 Suppl):188-202

[21] Wong RL, Hiyari S, Yaghsezian A, Davar M, Lin YL, Galvan M, et al. Comparing the healing potential of late-stage periodontitis and Peri-Implantitis. The Journal of Oral Implantology. 2017;**43**(6):437-445

[22] Maruyama N, Maruyama F, Takeuchi Y, Aikawa C, Izumi Y, Nakagawa I. Intraindividual variation in core microbiota in peri-implantitis and periodontitis. Scientific Reports. 2014;**4**:6602

[23] Zitzmann NU, Berglundh T, Ericsson I, Lindhe J. Spontaneous progression of experimentally induced periimplantitis. Journal of Clinical Periodontology. 2004;**31**(10):845-849

[24] Charalampakis G, Abrahamsson I, Carcuac O, Dahlen G, Berglundh T. Microbiota in experimental periodontitis and peri-implantitis in dogs. Clinical Oral Implants Research. 2013

[25] Marsh PD. Microbial ecology of dental plaque and its significance in health and disease. Advances in Dental Research. 1994;**8**(2):263-271

[26] Marsh PD. Are dental diseases examples of ecological catastrophes? Microbiology. 2003;**149**(2):279-294

[27] Heuer W, Elter C, Demling A, Neumann A, Suerbaum S, Hannig M, Heidenblut T, Bach FW, Stiesch-Scholz M. Analysis of early biofilm formation on oral implants in man. Journal of Oral Rehabilitation 2007;**34**(5):377-82

[28] Quirynen M, Vogels R, Pauwels M, Haffajee AD, Socransky SS, Uzel NG, et al. Initial subgingival colonization of 'pristine' pockets. Journal of Dental Research. 2005;**84**(4):340-344

[29] WA J, GR J, Claudia B, Tiddo F. Early colonization of dental implants by putative periodontal pathogens in partially edentulous patients. Clinical Oral Implants Research. 2000;**11**(6):511-520

[30] Griffen AL, Beall CJ, Firestone ND, Gross EL, DiFranco JM, Hardman JH, et al. CORE: A Phylogenetically-curated 16S rDNA database of the Core oral microbiome. PLoS One. 2011;**6**(4):e19051

[31] Costalonga M, Herzberg MC. The oral microbiome and the immunobiology of periodontal disease and caries. Immunology Letters. 2014;**162**(2 0 0):22-38

[32] Zaura E, Keijser BJF, Huse SM, Crielaard W. Defining the healthy "core microbiome" of oral microbial communities. BMC Microbiology. 2009;**9**:259

[33] Valente NA, Andreana S. Peri-implant disease: What we know and what we need to know. Journal of Periodontal & Implant Science. 2016;**46**(3):136-151

[34] Apse P, Ellen RP, Overall CM, Zarb GA. Microbiota and crevicular fluid collagenase activity in the osseointegrated dental implant sulcus: A comparison of sites in edentulous and partially edentulous patients. Journal of Periodontal Research. 1989;**24**(2):96-105

[35] Leonhardt A, Adolfsson B, Lekholm U, Wikstrom M, Dahlen G. A longitudinal microbiological study on osseointegrated titanium implants in partially edentulous patients. Clinical Oral Implants Research. 1993;**4**(3):113-120

[36] Quiryen M, Listgarten MA. The distribution of bacterial morphotypes around natural teeth and titanium implants ad modum Brånemark. Clinical Oral Implants Research. 1990;**1**(1):8-12

[37] Mombelli A, Decaillet F. The characteristics of biofilms in peri-implant disease. Journal of Clinical Periodontology. 2011;**38**(11 Suppl):203-213

[38] Carcuac O, Derks J, Charalampakis G, Abrahamsson I, Wennstrom J, Berglundh T. Adjunctive systemic and local antimicrobial therapy in the surgical treatment of Peri-implantitis: A randomized controlled clinical trial. Journal of Dental Research. 2015

[39] Charalampakis G, Belibasakis GN. Microbiome of peri-implant infections: Lessons from conventional, molecular and metagenomic analyses. Virulence. 2015;**6**(3):183-187

[40] Dabdoub SM, Tsigarida AA, Kumar PS. Patient-specific analysis of periodontal and Peri-implant microbiomes. Journal of Dental Research. 2013;**92**(12_suppl):168S-175S

[41] Kumar PS, Mason MR, Brooker MR, O'Brien K. Pyrosequencing reveals unique microbial signatures associated with healthy and failing dental implants. Journal of Clinical Periodontology. 2012;**39**(5):425-433

[42] Griffen AL, Beall CJ, Campbell JH, Firestone ND, Kumar PS, Yang ZK, et al. Distinct and complex bacterial profiles in human periodontitis and health revealed by 16S pyrosequencing. The Isme Journal. 2011;**6**:1176

[43] Abusleme L, Dupuy AK, Dutzan N, Silva N, Burleson JA, Strausbaugh LD, et al. The subgingival microbiome in health and periodontitis and its relationship with community biomass and inflammation. The Isme Journal. 2013;**7**:1016

[44] Lafaurie GI, Sabogal MA, Castillo DM, Rincon MV, Gomez LA, Lesmes YA, et al. Microbiome and microbial biofilm profiles of Peri-Implantitis: A systematic review. Journal of Periodontology. 2017;**88**(10):1066-1089

[45] Padial-Molina M, López-Martínez J, O'Valle F, Galindo-Moreno P. Microbial Profiles and Detection techniques in Peri-implant diseases: A systematic review. Journal of Oral & Maxillofacial Research. 2016;**7**(3):e10

[46] Leonhardt Å, Renvert S, Dahlén G. Microbial findings at failing implants. Clinical Oral Implants Research. 1999;**10**(5):339-345

[47] Albertini M, López-Cerero L, O'Sullivan MG, Chereguini CF, Ballesta S, Ríos V, et al. Assessment of periodontal and opportunistic flora in patients with peri-implantitis. Clinical Oral Implants Research. 2015;**26**(8):937-941

[48] Botero JE, González AM, Mercado RA, Olave G, Contreras A. Subgingival microbiota in Peri-implant mucosa lesions and adjacent teeth in partially edentulous patients. Journal of Periodontology. 2005;**76**(9):1490-1495

[49] Salvi GE, Fürst MM, Lang NP, Persson GR. One-year bacterial colonization patterns of Staphylococcus aureus and other bacteria at implants and adjacent teeth. Clinical Oral Implants Research. 2008;**19**(3):242-248

[50] Fürst MM, Salvi GE, Lang NP, Persson GR. Bacterial colonization immediately after installation on oral titanium implants. Clinical Oral Implants Research. 2007;**18**(4):501-508

[51] Al-Radha ASD, Pal A, Pettemerides AP, Jenkinson HF. Molecular analysis of microbiota associated with peri-implant diseases. Journal of Dentistry. 2012;**40**(11):989-998

[52] Apatzidou D, Lappin DF, Hamilton G, Papadopoulos CA, Konstantinidis A, Riggio MP. Microbiome of peri-implantitis affected and healthy dental sites in patients with a history of chronic periodontitis. Archives of Oral Biology. 2017;**83**:145-152

[53] Shibli JA, Melo L, Ferrari DS, Figueiredo LC, Faveri M, Feres M. Composition of supra- and subgingival biofilm of subjects with healthy and diseased implants. Clinical Oral Implants Research. 2008;**19**(10):975-982

[54] Zheng H, Xu L, Wang Z, Li L, Zhang J, Zhang Q, et al. Subgingival microbiome in patients with healthy and ailing dental implants. Scientific Reports. 2015;**5**:10948

[55] Koyanagi T, Sakamoto M, Takeuchi Y, Maruyama N, Ohkuma M, Izumi Y. Comprehensive microbiological findings in peri-implantitis and periodontitis. Journal of Clinical Periodontology. 2013;**40**(3):218-226

[56] Tamura NOM, Miyakawa H, Nakazawa F. Analysis of bacterial flora associated with peri-implantitis using obligate anaerobic culture technique and 16S rDNA gene sequence. The International Journal of Oral & Maxillofacial Implants. 2013;**28**(6):1521-1529

[57] da Silva ESC, Feres M, Figueiredo LC, Shibli JA, Ramiro FS, Faveri M. Microbiological diversity of peri-implantitis biofilm by sanger sequencing. Clinical Oral Implants Research. 2014;**25**(10):1192-1199

[58] Ebadian AR, Kadkhodazadeh M, Zarnegarnia P, Dahlén G. Bacterial analysis of Peri-implantitis and chronic periodontitis in Iranian subjects. Acta Medica Iranica. 2012:7

[59] Casado PL, Otazu IB, Balduino A, de Mello W, Barboza EP, Duarte MEL. Identification of periodontal pathogens in healthy Periimplant sites. Implant Dentistry. 2011;**20**(3):226-235

[60] Canullo L, Peñarrocha-Oltra D, Covani U, Botticelli D, Serino G, Penarrocha M. Clinical and microbiological findings in patients with peri-implantitis: A cross-sectional study. Clinical Oral Implants Research. 2016;**27**(3):376-382

[61] Hultin M, Gustafsson A, Hallstrom H, Johansson LA, Ekfeldt A, Klinge B. Microbiological findings and host response in patients with peri-implantitis. Clinical Oral Implants Research. 2002;**13**(4):349-358

[62] Cortelli SC, Cortelli JR, Romeiro RL, Costa FO, Aquino DR, Orzechowski PR, et al. Frequency of periodontal pathogens in equivalent peri-implant and periodontal clinical statuses. Archives of Oral Biology. 2013;**58**(1):67-74

[63] Ata-Ali J, Flichy-Fernández AJ, Alegre-Domingo T, Ata-Ali F, Palacio J, Peñarrocha-Diago M. Clinical, microbiological, and immunological aspects of healthy versus peri-implantitis tissue in full arch reconstruction patients: A prospective cross-sectional study. BMC Oral Health. 2015;**15**(1):43

[64] Wang H-L, Garaicoa-Pazmino C, Collins A, Ong H-S, Chudri R, Giannobile WV. Protein biomarkers and microbial profiles in peri-implantitis. Clinical Oral Implants Research. 2016;**27**(9):1129-1136

[65] Zhuang L-F, Watt RM, Mattheos N, Si M-S, Lai H-C, Lang NP. Periodontal and peri-implant microbiota in patients with healthy and inflamed periodontal and peri-implant tissues. Clinical Oral Implants Research. 2016;**27**(1):13-21

[66] Eick S, Ramseier CA, Rothenberger K, Brägger U, Buser D, Salvi GE. Microbiota at teeth and implants in partially edentulous patients. A 10-year retrospective study. Clinical Oral Implants Research. 2016;**27**(2):218-225

[67] Verdugo F, Castillo A, Simonian K, Russo P, D'Addona A, Raffaelli L, et al. Periodontopathogen and Epstein-Barr virus contamination affects transplanted bone volume in sinus augmentation. Journal of Periodontology. 2012;**83**(2):162-173

[68] Canullo LPP, Botticelli D, Covani U, Jankovic S, Jovanovic T, Rakic M. What is the impact of Epstein-Barr virus in Peri-implant infection? The International Journal of Oral & Maxillofacial Implants. 2018;**33**(1):58-63

[69] Belibasakis GN, Mir-Mari J, Sahrmann P, Sanz-Martin I, Schmidlin PR, Jung RE. Clinical association of Spirochaetes and Synergistetes with peri-implantitis. Clinical Oral Implants Research. 2016;**27**(6):656-661

[70] Koyanagi T, Sakamoto M, Takeuchi Y, Ohkuma M, Izumi Y. Analysis of microbiota associated with peri-implantitis using 16S rRNA gene clone library. Journal of Oral Microbiology. 2010;**2**(1):5104

[71] Yu X-L, Chan Y, Zhuang L-F, Lai H-C, Lang NP, Lacap-Bugler DC, et al. Distributions of Synergistetes in clinically-healthy and diseased periodontal and peri-implant niches. Microbial Pathogenesis. 2016;**94**:90-103

[72] Al-Ahmad A, Muzafferiy F, Anderson AC, Wolber JP, Ratka-Kruger P, Fretwurst T, et al. Shift of microbial composition of peri-implantitis-associated oral biofilm as revealed by 16S rRNA gene cloning. Journal of Medical Microbiology. 2018;**67**(3):332-340

[73] Tsigarida AA, Dabdoub SM, Nagaraja HN, Kumar PS. The influence of smoking on the Peri-implant microbiome. Journal of Dental Research. 2015;**94**(9):1202-1217

[74] Group TNHW, Peterson J, Garges S, Giovanni M, McInnes P, Wang L, et al. The NIH human microbiome project. Genome Research. 2009;**19**(12):2317-2323

[75] Frank JA, Reich CI, Sharma S, Weisbaum JS, Wilson BA, Olsen GJ. Critical evaluation of two primers commonly used for amplification of bacterial 16S rRNA genes. Applied and Environmental Microbiology. 2008;**74**(8):2461-2470

[76] DeLong EF, Preston CM, Mincer T, Rich V, Hallam SJ, Frigaard N-U, et al. Community genomics among stratified microbial assemblages in the Ocean's interior. Science. 2006; **311**(5760):496-503

[77] Streit WR, Schmitz RA. Metagenomics – The key to the uncultured microbes. Current Opinion in Microbiology. 2004;**7**(5):492-498

[78] Rams TE, Degener JE, van Winkelhoff AJ. Antibiotic resistance in human peri-implantitis microbiota. Clinical Oral Implants Research. 2014;**25**(1):82-90

[79] Verdugo F, Castillo A, Simonian K, Castillo F, Farez-Vidal E, D'Addona A. Periodontopathogen and Epstein–Barr virus-associated Periapical periodontitis may be the source of retrograde infectious Peri-Implantitis. Clinical Implant Dentistry and Related Research. 2015;**17**(1):199-207

[80] Heitz-Mayfield LJ, Salvi GE, Mombelli A, Faddy M, Lang NP, Implant Complication Research G. Anti-infective surgical therapy of peri-implantitis. A 12-month prospective clinical study. Clinical Oral Implants Research. 2012;**23**(2):205-210

[81] van Winkelhoff AJ, Wolf JW. Actinobacillus actinomycetemcomitans-associated peri-implantitis in an edentulous patient. A case report. Journal of Clinical Periodontology. 2000;**27**(7):531-535

[82] Leonhardt A, Dahlen G, Renvert S. Five-year clinical, microbiological, and radiological outcome following treatment of peri-implantitis in man. Journal of Periodontology. 2003;**74**(10):1415-1422

[83] Serino G, Turri A. Outcome of surgical treatment of peri-implantitis: Results from a 2-year prospective clinical study in humans. Clinical Oral Implants Research. 2011; **22**(11):1214-1220

[84] Khoury F, Buchmann R. Surgical therapy of peri-implant disease: A 3-year follow-up study of cases treated with 3 different techniques of bone regeneration. Journal of Periodontology. 2001;**72**(11):1498-1508

[85] Emrani J, Chee W, Slots J. Bacterial colonization of oral implants from nondental sources. Clinical Implant Dentistry and Related Research. 2009;**11**(2):106-112

[86] Mombelli A, Lang NP. Antimicrobial treatment of peri-implant infections. Clinical Oral Implants Research. 1992;**3**(4):162-168

[87] Roos-Jansåker A-M, Renvert H, Lindahl C, Renvert S. Surgical treatment of peri-implantitis using a bone substitute with or without a resorbable membrane: A prospective cohort study. Journal of Clinical Periodontology. 2007;**34**(7):625-632

[88] Claffey N, Clarke E, Polyzois I, Renvert S. Surgical treatment of peri-implantitis. Journal of Clinical Periodontology. 2008;**35**(8 Suppl):316-332

[89] Poveda Roda R, Bagán JV, Sanchis Bielsa JM, Carbonell Pastor E. Antibiotic Use in Dental Practice: A Review. Medicina Oral, Patología Oral Y Cirugía Bucal (Internet). 2007;**12**:186-192

[90] Sullivan A, Edlund C, Nord CE. Effect of antimicrobial agents on the ecological balance of human microflora. The Lancet Infectious Diseases. 2001;**1**(2):101-114

[91] Rashid MU, Weintraub A, Nord CE. Effect of new antimicrobial agents on the ecological balance of human microflora. Anaerobe. 2012;**18**(2):249-253

[92] Nord CE. Studies on the ecological impact of antibiotics. European Journal of Clinical Microbiology & Infectious Diseases. 1990;**9**(7):517-518

[93] Van der Waaij D, Nord CE. Development and persistence of multi-resistance to antibiotics in bacteria; an analysis and a new approach to this urgent problem. International Journal of Antimicrobial Agents. 2000;**16**(3):191-197

[94] Verdugo F, Laksmana T, Uribarri A. Systemic antibiotics and the risk of superinfection in peri-implantitis. Archives of Oral Biology. 2016;**64**:39-50

[95] Teles FRF. The microbiome of Peri-implantitis: Is it unique? The Compendium of Continuing Education in Dentistry. 2017;**38**:22-25